Handbook
of
Voice Therapy
for the
School Clinician

HANDBOOK
OF
VOICE THERAPY
FOR THE
SCHOOL CLINICIAN

William R. Leith
Robert G. Johnston

Taylor & Francis Ltd
London

Published by
Taylor & Francis Ltd, 4 John Street, London WC1N 2ET

First published by College-Hill Press, 4284 41 St., San Diego, California 92105

Library of Congress Cataloging-in-Publication Data
Main entry under title:

Leith, William, 1927–
    Handbook of voice therapy for the school clinician.

    Includes index.
    1. Voice disorders in children—Treatment. I. Johnston, Robert G.,
1942–   . II. Title. [DNLM: 1. Voice Disorders—in infancy & child-
hood. 2. Voice Disorders—therapy. WM 475 L533ha]
    RF511.5.C45L45   1986   618.92'855   86-6152

ISBN 0-316-520403

British Library Cataloguing in Publication Data

Leith, William R.
    Handbook of voice therapy for the school clinician.
    1. Speech therapy for children
    I. Title II. Johnston, Robert G.
618.92'85506   LB3454

ISBN 0-85066-607-4

This edition not for sale in the American continent

Printed in the United States of America

*To all clinicians who are providing therapy
for persons who have voice disorders and
to all persons who have voice disorders
who are receiving therapy*

CONTENTS

SECTION II: THE PRETHERAPY PROCESS

SECTION III: THE THERAPY PROCESS

PREFACE

From the hundreds if not thousands of school clinicians we have talked to about our profession we hear a relatively constant theme, that of being uncomfortable doing therapy in the areas of stuttering and voice disorders. We can appreciate the discomfort with stuttering, since there are so many theories and therapies that do not work; that is, they do not eliminate the stuttering, and the clinician is clinically frustrated.

We are also sympathetic with the clinican's frustration over voice therapy. It is not so much that there are so many theories and therapy that it is difficult to settle on one approach, it is that there are so many divergent views of the same problem and, regardless of the view, they all use the same basic therapy. It is indeed confusing when one person views a specific disorder as a hoarse voice whereas another person, viewing the exact same disorder, discusses it from the standpoint of vocal abuse, and still a third views the situation from the standpoint of excess tension in the larynx. So, which way do we turn? Do we settle on the auditorily oriented descriptive terms we can not define, or do we settle on medical problems over which we have no jurisdiction, or do we attempt to estimate degrees of tension we cannot observe? And, when we make our decision, what do we do about therapy? These views do not deal with the remediation of the disorder; they are only descriptive terms or etiological classifications. Is it any wonder that clinicians are confused?

Having taught courses in voice disorders for many years, we were also confused. If we selected a textbook that was medically oriented, then a good share of the course time was spent on teaching about laryngeal diseases and viewing slides of laryngeal pathology. But, in reality, the students were never to be involved in the medical aspects of vocal disorders. If there was a pathologic condition, the medical community took care of it and only then did the speech clinician evaluate the person to see if there were any residual effects.

On the other hand, if we selected a text that was oriented to the auditory descriptive label so often applied to voice disorders, such as hoarse, breathy, and harsh, we spent a lot of time having our students listening to tape recordings of the various types of voices. However, this picture was usually clouded by the tapes describing the voice disorders both auditorily and medically, such as hoarse voice due to vocal nodes or breathy voice due to laryngeal paralysis. Sometimes it got totally out of hand when the first voice sample was hoarseness due to polyps and the second sample was hoarseness due to laryngeal paralysis. And what did our students say to all this? "Whoa! You mean a hoarse voice can be associated with either added mass like nodes or polyps or with flaccid folds like with paralysis?" No doubt about it. When viewed from these standpoints, voice therapy is a very confusing area.

The planning of this book started 2 years ago. The more we talked about voice therapy the more we became convinced that the only logical approach to vocal disorders was the behavioral approach. Building on the cognitive behavior therapy model presented in the first two books in this handbook series, the behavioral approach to voice disorders was developed. It is a system that we feel is very logical, easy to comprehend, and applicable in any clinical setting. We feel secure in the behavioral approach to voice therapy and we hope that you find clinical security with voice disorders in this book.

William R. Leith
Robert G. Johnston

ACKNOWLEDGMENTS

We want to thank all of the speech-language clinicians in the schools in metropolitan areas of Detroit and Cleveland who have worked on this and the other two books in this series, *Handbook of Clinical Methods in Communication Disorders* and *Handbook of Stuttering Therapy for the School Clinician,* over the years to make certain that they realistically address the unique clinical problems faced in the school environment. Our thanks also to the many programs and agencies that allowed us to do workshops in voice therapy so we could test our presentation of our concepts and treatment procedures. We would also like to thank Dr. Mae Taylor, Specialist in Communication Disorders with the Utah State Board of Education, for her special assistance. Very special thanks to all of the students at Wayne State University who took the graduate course in voice disorders; they were very patient with the slow development of many of the concepts.

Finally, the first author wants to thank CVR for teaching him the importance of the clinician and therapy in his chosen profession.

Section I
Basic Information

Chapter 1

Introduction

VOICE AND SOCIETY

Disorders of voice present a special challenge to the speech/language pathologist. To begin, it is difficult even to decide what constitutes a voice disorder. What is a voice disorder? Let us start our discussion by consider the following telephone call:

Caller: Is this the Metropolitan Speech and Language Clinic?
Secretary: Yes it is. Can I help you?
Caller: I certainly hope so. My name is Smith. I am a senior in high school and I am having a problem with my voice.
Secretary: I am certain we can provide you with some help, Miss Smith. What seems to be the problem with your voice?
Caller: Well, for one thing, my name is Paul.

Does Paul have a voice problem? First and foremost, it depends on how he feels about it. If it does not bother him to be mistaken for a woman, then there really is no clinical voice problem. However, since he called the clinic requesting some help, we can assume that there is a clinical problem.

One thing clinicians must take into consideration when dealing with voice deviations is the social reaction to voice. Voices vary from those that are viewed as exceptional to those that annoy people. However, society is very lenient in terms of how far a voice deviates before it becomes a social, emotional, or economic handicap. It is only when the deviation creates social, emotional, or economic handicaps that it becomes a problem. We, as professionals, may judge a voice, saying in our most pontifical tones, "That individual has a voice problem." But what we are actually saying is that, in *our* judgment (which may not be very valid or reliable), the voice we are listening to deviates significantly from what we would consider "normal" or "average." This says nothing about how the voice is perceived by society. And, what would we do if the person whose voice we judged asked us what the "normal" or "average" voice is? They might embarrass us even more

—NOTES—

by asking us what the "normal" pitch level is, or how loud the "average" voice is, or what the "normal" quality is for a voice. There is no such thing as normal pitch, loudness, or quality of a voice. It all depends on how other people, society, if you will, views the voice. What we may consider an extremely deviant voice, ripe for therapy, society might view as a "most interesting" voice. If you think of the voices of some famous people, you will find some have what might be considered very poor voices. Yet there is no social penalty for the voice. In fact, in some instances, it is the deviant voice itself that is rewarded.

To carry this social influence in classification of vocal problem a bit further, the clinician must also recognize that social responses differ according to which parameter of voice is involved. Variations in the parameters of pitch and loudness often lead to stereotyping of the individual. For example, the male whose pitch is judged too high is considered to be feminine, whereas the female with a pitch that is too low is viewed as masculine. Persons who speak too soft are considered withdrawn or timid people, and others who speak too loud are boisterous or aggressive. When considering voice quality, there are so many possible variations that society does not seem to have many stereotypes. Generally speaking, the "breathy" voice is considered "sexy" by many people. The "harsh" voice is often associated by society with people who are aggressive and vindictive. And the "hoarse" voice is that of the Godfather. So much for overgeneralization. It may seem in our society that deviant voice qualities are admired because they are distinctive. Children often imitate unique voice qualities, such as that identified with "Popeye" or with some of the other characters in various cartoons, television shows, or movies. Deviant voices may indeed call attention to themselves and, as we all know, attention is often very positive, rewarding the very vocal parameter we are telling the client is creating a problem.

As can be seen, it is tenuous at best to say that a specific vocal pitch, loudness, or quality is a problem. It is difficult enough to say that it is a deviant voice (since we do not know what it deviates from), let alone to make a statement that it is creating problems for the individual. The best judge of when a voice is a problem is the person whose voice it is.

This creates a rather unique clinical problem with clients who have been determined to have voice disorders, that being, client motivation. Since society is so lenient in terms of vocal deviations, there is very little social rejection associated with vocal deviations. Children are teased about their "baby talk" or their stuttering, but you would be hard pressed to find children who were teased about their voices. The child whose voice was changing in puberty, producing vocal breaks, may be the point of teasing, and, perhaps, the rare instance of a child whose vocal pitch was so deviant that other children made fun of it may be seen, but these are the exception, not the rule. Consider also that if a child has a deviant voice quality, other children may attempt to imitate it, not to tease the child, but to learn to do it since it is distinctive.

If the voice creates no social problems, and there is no teasing, and there are no communication problems associated with the voice, why then would the client be motivated to work on changing his voice? In many instances he is not, but he is thrust into therapy because someone else has decided he should have it. The other person is almost always either the speech clinician or the child's parents. Voice problems do not carry the social stigma that other communication problems do. The clinician cannot rely on this as a motivational device with most clients. The problem of client motivation will be discussed in detail later in the book.

This sociological response to vocal deviation may partially explain why voice therapy is one of the most frustrating clinical areas the speech clinician faces. But in order to more fully understand the clinician's frustrations, we must dig a bit deeper into our professional philosophy and training in the treatment of voice disorders.

VOICE THERAPY: A CLINICIAN'S DILEMMA

Before embarking on this discussion, some terminology that will be used throughout the book will be clarified. Without attempting to defend the position, the speech/language clinician (speech clinician from this point on) will be referred to as "she" and the client will be referred to as "he." This may be sexist (Why is it that only males have voice disorders?), but it certainly helps with identifying who we are talking about. With this in mind, let us proceed. There appear to be three basic problems clinicians face when they attempt to learn to do voice therapy: the organization of the materials in voice texts, the lack of a clear rationale for the clinical approaches to the disorders, and the lack of clinical training.

Organization of Material

According to Pannbacker (1984), the current texts tend to organize themselves around three main classification themes. The most popular classification theme appears to be "auditory" classifications such as "hoarse," "breathy," and "harsh." In fact, with very few exceptions, these are the terms most often used in texts and voice evaluations to describe voice quality problems. Even references that have orientations other than acoustic also use these terms. Pannbacker (1984) lists 71 different terms that are used to describe voice quality. To appreciate the semantic problems here consider just three of the terms, breathy, harsh and hoarse, and see how four different authors view them.

Breathy

Moore, G. P. (1964): "Breathy voice quality is made up of the vocal fold sound plus whispered noise produced by audible turbulent air. . . . There is a ratio of breath noise to phonatory sound and this is what determines the quality of the breathy voice. . . . At one end of the continuum one hears predominantly the phonatory aspect while at the other end one hears the increased air flow and turbulence."

Wilson, P. K. (1979): "The characteristics of breathiness are whispered sounds, vocal cord tones that are weak, a noise element, limited range of vocal intensity, and low pitch. . . . There is a wide range of severity of breathiness, from mild to complete aphonia."

Murphy, A. T. (1964): "Breathiness is the presence of an excessive amount of breath accompanying the vocal tone. . . . In some breathiness there is no tone, just breath during speech attempt. . . . Some other terms used to describe breathiness are fuzzy, veiled, hoarse, whispered."

Van Riper, C. (1981): "Breathy voice quality is characterized by an excessive flow of air along with the phonation. . . . Breathy voices are not whispered but they do have aspirate quality."

Harsh

Moore, G. P. (1964): "A very low pitched voice that falls below the lowest part of the individual's phonatory range. . . a voice that contains popping or ticking components which are determined by the glottal pulses . . . a voice that has a 'roughness' component."

Wilson, D. K. (1979): "A voice that is unpleasant and rough and may contain some vocal fry . . . a voice that has a very low pitch . . . a voice that sounds constricted."

Murphy, A. T. (1964): "Harsh voices are usually characterized by a lower than normal pitch, but high pitched harsh voices also occur. . . . High pitched harsh voices are referred to as strident or metallic voices. . . . Many harsh voices also have excessive nasal resonance. . . .

Harsh voices are also described as strident, coarse, grating, rasping, rough, metallic, gutteral, harsh-strident, harsh-throaty."

Van Riper, C. (1981): "Harsh voices are characterized by vocal fry. . . . When the pitch of the vocal fry is high and there is tension, the voice is strident or harsh."

Hoarse

Moore, G. P. (1964): "Hoarseness is a combination of low pitched phonatory sounds and a noise component. . . . There is a great range in hoarse voices where the voice may appear similar to a breathy voice to a voice that is almost all noise. . . . In rough hoarseness one gets the impression of a second very low pitched sound being superimposed on the voice."

Wilson, D. K. (1979): "Hoarseness is a combination of harshness and breathiness. . . . The range of hoarse voices is due to the harsh element dominating in some voices and the breathiness dominating in others. . . . The voice is rough, somewhat discordant and low in pitch."

Murphy, A. T. (1964): "Hoarseness may be best thought of as breathy, husky harshness. . . . The pitch level of these voices is usually low. . . . The voice usually fluctuates between periods of phonation and periods of aphonia. . . . Hoarse voices are also described as breathy, harsh, raspy, strained, coarse, and hollow."

Van Riper, C. (1981): "Hoarseness is the result of a combination of breathy and harsh voice qualities."

As you can see, there are common themes running through the authors' definitions but the clinician can still easily become caught in a semantic trap with these terms. For example, the hoarse voice is said to be a combination of breathy and harsh voice quality. However, if you are not clear what a harsh voice is, you are really at a loss to describe a hoarse voice. A famous voice clinician, now retired from Purdue University, once said after examining a client, "That client's voice is hoarse enough to pull a wagon." This may not be a very professional assessment of the client's voice but it probably represents the views of many clinicians who struggle with the "auditory" approach to voice therapy. In addition, there is no clear or obvious voice therapy that relates to such classifications even if clinicians can agree on them.

Other voice texts are "disorder oriented"; that is, each disorder is identified according to its medical classification and a treatment program is then associated with the classified disorder. Reading one of these books is like reading a mystery story backwards. First you find

—NOTES—

out who did it and then you find out what they did. In the tradition of all good mystery stories, there are numerous suspects (disorders or diseases), they all appear at first glance to play some role in the crime (disappearance of good voice), most of the evidence presented is irrelevant, and unfortunately, most of the medical terminology remains a mystery even after the book is read. The reader must deal with such things as lesions, webs, stenosis, cysts, papillomas, inflamed tissue, disease, polyps, arthritis, tumors, glandular deficiencies, neurological disruptions, myoclonus, hyperkinesthesia, syndromes, apraxia, dysarthria, and so on. This is a whole new area of professional jargon.

The problem the clinician faces with this classification theme is to find a classification that perfectly reflects the disorder manifested by a client, and this is no mean task: this is the mystery. There are a multitude of vocal variations to each medical classification, and the clinician is often left with a disorder that seems to fit two classifications, or none at all. This approach to vocal problems can be viewed as a matching contest, a test to see if the clinician can find a classification that matches her client or to find a client whose vocal disorder matches a classification.

The final theme is the hyper/hypo function classification, based on the amount of tension present in the vocal folds. Pannbacker (1984) lists this as a kinesiologic classification system. It can also be viewed as a behaviorally oriented system, since judgments are made on assumed vocal performances rather than on medical problems or classification of the auditory signal. Its weakness, according to Aronson (1980) and Morris and Spriestersbach (1978), is that it is an oversimplification of the laryngeal system. Some writers have expanded this behavioral concept a bit by also considering the relationship of mass-size alterations of the vocal folds. Pannbacker (1984) points out a problem with this system in that conditions such as cord thickening that increase the mass of the folds also prevent their approximation.

Since voice courses are often planned around the text selected for the class, the organization of the textbooks influences the type of training students receive in various professional training programs. So speech clinicians have one of these three general orientations—auditory, disorder oriented, or hyper/hypo function. Talk about communication disorders! Consider what happens when two clinicians, one with a medical and the other with an auditory orientation, attempt to discuss a client with a voice disorder. It is reminiscent of the Tower of Babel. They find it almost impossible to communicate, since each has not only a different view of the same problem but also different vocabularies.

Clinical Rationale for Therapy

The second problem, the lack of a clear rationale for therapy procedures, seems related both to the type of communication disorder being dealt with as well as the organization of the textbooks. Let us discuss the influence of the type of disorder by contrasting therapy planning with an articulation case with that of a voice case. We have noted with interest that if a student clinician is assigned an articulation case, she wants to know what articulation behaviors are omitted, distorted, substituted, or added. She also wants to know the context in which the errors occur, the client's phonological rule system, and the effect of coarticulatory demands. She wants a great deal of behavioral information before she feels confident to plan her treatment procedure. To gather information, she applies numerous evaluative instruments and invests much clinical time in the evaluation process.

However, when assigned a voice problem, the student clinician seems more easily satisfied. About all the information she seems to want is a medical, auditory, or tension classification. The fact that the clinician does not request or seek additional behavioral information when confronted with a voice case may be the result of the particular approach to voice therapy that is presented in the various texts currently available. All that is needed is a medical diagnosis, an auditory term describing the voice, or some indication of vocal fold tension and she is in business. The clinician simply looks up the particular classification in the book and, low and behold, there is the therapy. She just follows the instructions and can alleviate the voice disorder. Too often, however, the book's classification system and the therapy approaches are seemingly unrelated.

With this kind of approach to voice therapy the clinician is not expected to understand the relationship between the "symptom" (medical, auditory, or tension) and the therapy. There is indeed a relationship between the therapy procedure and the medical etiology, but in most texts it is not spelled out; a therapy plan is simply "prescribed" for the clinician to follow. No explanation is necessary when you are given a "prescription" to take or follow. The medical model is followed closely in these texts. With the auditory classification, there is no relationship to understand. "Hoarse" voices can result from such a wide variety of etiological factors that there is no therapeutic implication with the label. Therapy planning will have to be based on some other factor, usually a subheading under "hoarse voice quality" having to do with an organic factor. But that, of course, is a "hoarse" of a different color.

—NOTES—

Clinical Training

Along with multiple classification themes and the lack of a clear rationale for therapy, there are also problems associated with clinical training in voice therapy. We should recognize that training in voice therapy has been historically associated with an apprenticeship model. This model was useful, particularly when the student had a "master" voice clinician available to demonstrate the therapy of choice with certain vocal disorders. More recently, the apprenticeship model was expanded to include a perceptual training/agreement process. This process attempted to quantify and objectify voice by way of scoring the attributes of what we perceived. Several authors made available audio tapes of abnormal voices, usually by disorder type, and a scoring procedure. The purpose of the tapes was to train the clinicians to recognize the sounds of vocal disorders. Although there remains a certain common sense usefulness in this approach, two problems remain. First, listener agreement is very difficult to obtain, particularly from tapes as opposed to live voices. Second, and more important, perceptual agreement does not in any way lead to therapy procedures that are appropriate for the client.

Even when the clinician can "correctly" identify a breathy, harsh, or hoarse voice, there is no direct relationship between the classification and the treatment procedure she looks up in a reference. She still is not provided with insights in the dynamics of the voice disorder and how these relate to the therapy procedure. Then, heaven forbid, if the therapy "recipe" does not resolve the problem, she is lost. She can not modify the treatment procedure in any logical way to meet the client's clinical needs, since she does not understand the rationale for the treatment.

In addition to these problems, we must also recognize the lack of clinical experience most clinicians have had in the area of voice disorders during their training. If they did have the opportunity to work with a voice client, he probably had been in therapy in the training clinic for several semesters and was more familiar with the therapy program than the clinicians. This is an unfortunate situation but there are very few training programs with a large enough case load in voice disorders to allow all the students to have diverse experience with voice cases. This lack of clinical experience also applies to the "on the job training" all clinicians receive. When the clinician first enters the profession, how much experience does she get with voice disorders? Very little: The incidence of voice disorders is quite low. This is not because of the lack of deviant voices but because society does not deem most of them a handicap. We, as clinicians, hear many voices we feel are in need of clinical modification. However, as was pointed out earlier in this chapter, it is society that determines vocal handicaps, not the ear of a clinician.

So, to summarize the clinical situation in voice therapy, the clinician enters the profession usually having had only one course dealing with voice disorders. Further, the course was probably either medically or auditorally oriented, giving no rationale for therapy, only recipes that are difficult to follow. Finally, the clinician enters the profession with very little supervised clinical experience with voice disorders. Under these conditions it is no wonder most clinicians would rather not work with clients who have voice disorders.

BEHAVIORAL APPROACH TO VOICE THERAPY

This book represents an attempt to provide the clinician with a handbook of voice therapy that is both understandable and practical. The nontraditional (but certainly not novel) approach to the treatment of voice disorders presented in this book should help in the understanding of this troublesome clinical area. However, the behavioral approach may pose some problems for the reader who has had extensive traditional training in voice disorders, since this book is not organized around auditory labels or medical classifications. Nor are we going to be vitally interested in attempting to estimate the amount of tension present in the larynx. However, we are vitally concerned with an *appropriate* assessment of the vocal problem. In our opinion, inappropriate assessments that are not directly related to the treatment program are the major stumbling block in providing adequate services to clients with vocal disorders.

We will be viewing voice disorders from the standpoint of what vocal behaviors the client can or cannot perform and how this behavioral performance (or lack of it) is reflected in the total vocal performance. It is the client's inability to perform various vocal behaviors that results in his voice disorders. His inability to perform the vocal behaviors may or may not be due to a medical or structural problem. Regardless of the reason the vocal behaviors are absent or distorted, it is the absence or distortion of the vocal behaviors themselves that constitute the vocal disorder.

As various vocal behavior problems are discussed, some terminology that is traditionally associated with voice disorders will be used, such as "hoarse," "breathy," "vocal nodes," and so forth. However, this usage is only to supplement the behavioral information, not to create a base or rationale for treatment. The behavioral approach does

—NOTES—

not discard or reject all of the current or historic information on voice disorders. Rather, we will construct our rationale for treatment of various vocal behavioral disorders by building on and expanding existing information.

Competence/Performance Behavioral Evaluation

During the past two decades our profession has begun to identify itself with a competence/performance model. In this model we compare a client's behavioral performance with what is considered to be normal performance. However, we cannot determine if something is "abnormal" until we determine what "normal" is. This means that we must gather enough data to establish what constitutes "normal" performance. Once this is accomplished, we then have a "standard" to compare with the client's performance. When behavioral incompetence has been determined, therapy can be planned to focus on those behaviors. The construct that supports the competence/performance evaluation is that the better we are able to understand how the normal system works, the better we will understand the abnormal system and how to remediate it.

What is a competence/performance based voice evaluation? It is the assessment of specific vocal behaviors performed by a client to determine if the performances fall within what is perceived to be normal limits. The focus of Chapter 3 is on how the normal vocal system works and the behavioral performances that are associated with normal vocal competence. In addition, even though we currently have inadequate normative data on vocal competence, we can expect the vocal system to perform certain specific behaviors and can have reasonable judgment of what constitutes normal performance. Further, armed with our knowledge of how the normal vocal system works and how aerodynamic principles govern the system, we can make several assumptions on how certain abnormal vocal systems will perform.

A competence/performance based voice evaluation is the logical application of accepted information on laryngeal anatomy, physiology, mechanics, and aerodynamics into a systematic evaluation. The client is asked to perform several vocal behaviors ranging from simple to complex, and the clinician evaluates the client's performances. From these performances the clinician makes judgments about the client's vocal competence. These competency judgments lead the clinician to a prescriptivelike approach to resolving the vocal problem; a one-to-one relationship develops between what is evaluated and what is remediated.

Thus, the voice evaluation in this clinical approach differs from the more traditional evaluations. We are not focusing on a auditory or medical classification of the voice disorder. We are attempting to determine why the vocal system cannot produce normal voice; that is, which vocal behaviors necessary for normal voice are not being performed adequately. We will then determine why the behaviors are not occurring and what we can do about them in therapy.

Cognitive Behavior Therapy

The cognitive behavior therapy that is introduced in this book is an important extension of what might be viewed as pure behavior therapy. It has all the advantages of behavior therapy, a systematic approach to behavioral disorders and a focus on behavioral events whose occurrences can be evaluated, but it also has the advantage of utilizing the client's cognitive processes in therapy. All clients *think* during therapy, and if the client is thinking of things other than your therapy, your therapy will lose some of its effectiveness. So, if we acknowledge that thinking is occurring during our therapy, and we guide what the client is thinking about, we can use the cognitive process to assist our therapy rather than detract from it. This is cognitive behavior therapy. It is a systematic and lawful approach to communication disorders, voice disorders in this case. The therapy is based on behavioral performance data to determine the behavior change goal and on learning theory to teach a new or modify an existing vocal behavior. The concepts involved in cognitive behavior therapy will be presented in the next chapter.

Vocal Behaviors

Thus far in this chapter we have talked about vocal behavior in a rather general way; that is, we have not mentioned any specific behavioral events and labeled them as vocal behaviors. We will present and discuss specific vocal behaviors in detail in Chapter 3. However, as we conclude this orientation to the behavioral approach to voice therapy, let us consider some behavioral categories that we include under the general heading of vocal behaviors. We include, as vocal behaviors, all behaviors involved in providing the energy necessary for vocalization. Essentially, this would include respiration and checking action during exhalation. We can generally refer to this category of behaviors as "respiration," remembering to include checking action.

The next grouping of behaviors would be those that actually generate the acoustic signal, the voice, which we will categorize as "phonation." However, there are a number of independent behaviors involved

—NOTES—

in this categorization. For example, there is a laryngeal behavior that results in approximation of the vocal folds and another that opens the approximated vocal folds. There is also the aerodynamic behavior of the vocal folds, proper synchronous vibration for clear tonal quality. We must also consider the stability of these behaviors over time. If the vocal folds occasionally close spasmodically or they vary from synchronized to unsynchronized vibration, this lack of stability is an important behavior.

Continuing with "phonatory," or laryngeal behaviors, we must also consider behaviors resulting in changes in length, tension, mass, and compression of the vocal folds. These changes influence the pitch, loudness, and prosody of the voice. We must remember that the behaviors involved in changing pitch and in changing loudness are independent behaviors. In other words, a person can change the pitch of the voice without changing loudness, or vice versa. The behaviors are also inseparable in that if there is no pitch, there is no voice, and if there is no loudness, there is no voice. It is the interaction of these behaviors that provide the voice with prosody.

The final behavioral category is that of "resonance." Resonance itself is an acoustic phenomenon, but we are interested in the vocal behavior that allows certain types of resonance to occur. There are many acoustic factors and variables that can be considered under the heading of "resonance," but we limit ourselves to one behavior and one acoustic phenomenon: the behavior of the nasopharyngeal port and the resultant role of nasal resonance in the voice.

The human voice is a thing of beauty when it is properly presented. When it cannot be produced normally, it presents an exciting challenge to the clinician. Perhaps we are bordering on the realm of aesthetics, but the voice can be a valuable asset or a serious liability, and you, the speech clinician, can be instrumental in changing a liability into an asset. Enjoy your challenge!

Chapter 2

Cognitive Behavior Therapy

THE COGNITIVE BEHAVIORAL ORIENTATION

The following presentation of the principles of cognitive behavior therapy is in an abbreviated form. The detailed presentation of this approach to therapy is contained in the book *Handbook of Clinical Methods in Communication Disorders*, by Leith (1984). Cognitive behavior therapy is the core of the voice treatment program presented here and it is strongly recommended that you review the material contained in the aforementioned reference for a more comprehensive understanding of the concept.

As we discuss the development and treatment of vocal disorders we will consider both cognitive and behavioral factors. Our cognitive behavior therapy will utilize concepts from both cognitive learning systems as well as from operant conditioning. It is important that we recognize the interaction between cognitive learning and "noncognitive" conditioning and that the client's cognitions, his thinking processes, are an integral part of the therapy process and may well be involved in the development of the vocal problem. The cognitive and behavioral influence in the development of vocal problems will be discussed in chapters to follow. In this chapter we will develop the concepts involved in our cognitive behavior therapy.

Cognitive behavior modification, as a specialized area of behavior therapy, was introduced in the late 1970s by Meichenbaum (1977). There are references listed in the References and Recommended Readings section for further study in this area. In our discussions of the role of cognition in therapy, we will consider the cognitive involvement both of the client and of the clinician. The client must perceive and comprehend all of the information presented to him by the clinician. The clinician must also be involved in therapy on a cognitive level; evaluating the client's responses, determining an appropriate response to the client's behavior, changing the clinical strategy if the client fails to respond or comprehend, and so forth. With some vocal disorders, the clinician must be aware of the client's cognitive set (that is, his atti-tudes, emotions, feelings, and needs). With these clients, the cognitive set is an important part of therapy and is used in each phase of therapy.

We will start our discussion of our cognitive behavior therapy by considering some basic learning theories and concepts. However, before we discuss them, it is important that we clarify some of the terminol-ogy we will be using. In operant conditioning, the terms *reinforce* and *punish* may be confusing to some and create misunderstanding in others. This is particularly true of *punish*. The terms *reward* and *penalty* are often used as synonyms for *reinforce* and *punish*. These are the terms we will use as we discuss operant procedures, since the terms are clearer in mean-ing to people not familiar with operant conditioning. This is an impor-tant consideration for the school clinician, who must communicate with other professionals such as administrators, teachers, occupational ther-apists, physical therapists, and counselors, who may not have a clear understanding of *reinforce* and *punish*. The term *punish* has negative connotations. The term *penalize* does not seem to have the same degree of negative impact.

When we apply a reward or a penalty, we create different attitudes in our clients, different clinical cognitive sets. With a reward, the client's attitude is positive and he performs those behaviors that yield more rewards. When penalty is used, the client's attitude is negative in that he avoids performing the behavior that results in penalty. He will per-form some other behavior so he will not be penalized. These different cognitive sets are very important, because we will be using both in our therapy. In order to identify them we will use the terms *approach moti-vation* and *avoidance motivation*.

When a client's behavior is followed by something positive (a reward), the client acquires *approach motivation*. He is motivated to perform the behavior more often in order to achieve more of the reward. If the client's behavior is followed by something negative (a penalty), the client acquires *avoidance motivation*. He is motivated to avoid the penalty by not performing the behavior as often. We are now ready to discuss two of the more important learning concepts.

LEARNING SYSTEMS

Our treatment program will utilize concepts and principles primar-ily from three learning approaches, cognitive, motor, and behavioral. We will discuss each rather briefly and then refer the reader to additional references for a broader and deeper understanding of the approaches.

Cognitive Learning

Cognition is a complex phenomenon. It is involved in receiving of information, thinking about the information, and planning the response to the information. Those aspects of cognition most important to the speech clinician are memory and problem solving.

The two types of memory are long term and short term memory. Long term memory implies that information is retained over long periods of time. In order for it to be retained, it must be rehearsed often; recitation of your name and telephone number is one such example. Remembering information you received in a class during your training might be another. You may have remembered it long enough to pass tests, but do you still remember it? It depends on how often you use it and recall it. If the information is not recalled periodically, it is "forgotten." A good example of this might be the vocal anatomy and physiology you were taught in your training program. How well would you do on an exam right now?

Short term memory is for information to be retained briefly and then discarded. It is our short term memory that allows us to remember a telephone number long enough to dial it, or to remember the names of people at social functions, or (with some of us) where we parked our car in a parking structure.

We use both forms of memory in our therapy. When we teach a new behavior or concept, we depend on the client remembering this for an extended period of time. The lack of long term memory creates problems in our therapy. If the client does not remember things from one therapy session to the next, each clinical session must start from the beginning of therapy, with each session being a new experience for the client.

Short term memory also has an impact on therapy. We often give our clients instructions for performing a task or a behavior. If this information is not retained long enough to influence the performance of the task or behavior, we have a serious problem in providing therapy.

Memory is also the source of problems with the cognitive set of some of our clients, their attitudes, beliefs, emotions, concepts, and so forth. These clients become emotionally involved with their vocal problems, sensitive to the embarrassment and to the penalties they receive. They develop a negative cognitive set based on these memo-

—NOTES—

ries, and this set becomes a very important factor in therapy with these clients.

Another aspect of cognition that influences therapy is problem solving through insight. This is the recognition of a solution to a problem. It is the sudden realization of the relationships between factors or bits of information. There is a word game that is based on problem solving through insight. Examine the following word games and see of you can solve the problem. We will give the answers at the end of the chapter.

1. PIT CH
2. TENVOCALSITY
3. *GLOTTAL*

   AIR PRESSURE

We present our clients with "problems" to which they must find solutions. For example, we model a behavior and they must find a way to imitate it. We give them information on how to change the quality of the voice, and they have to figure out how to do it. They must integrate all this information, see the interrelationships, and gain insight into the "problem" before they can produce the behavior correctly. Consider the client who is given the rules concerning phonology. He must "understand" the rules before he can apply them to his speech. In other words, he must see the relationships between the rules and his speech (gain "insight") before there is a change in the speech or vocal behaviors.

We might view this as verbal comprehension. Our client can only comprehend what we tell him after he has compared this with his long term memories of past experiences and understands the relationships between what we said and what he has experienced. He must understand not only the words he hears, but also the relationships between them and the concepts they convey.

In that therapy with these clients deals with a structure—the larynx—that is normally not directly under voluntary control and is not visible, our models of behavior and information on how to perform a behavior cannot be directly applied by the client. He must accomplish the new behavior by judging its correctness after his attempt to imitate the model, which is influenced by his lack of direct muscular control over the larynx. Contrast this with the client attempting to produce a phoneme; whose production can be seen. Not only is the client able to see and hear the model, he also has voluntary control over his articulators. There is a relatively direct cognitive route between the sensory input and the imitative motor output. This is not the case with the voice client. He may indeed receive the same amount of information about the desired behavior, but there is no direct cognitive route to the motor output; it is reflexive in nature. This tends to explain why the clinician has difficulty teaching more appropriate vocal fold closure, easy vocal onset, and so on.

Sometimes the clinician must move away from models and information of behaviors and utilize existent behaviors that, when performed, precipitate the desired behavior to occur. For example, how would the clinician teach the client to produce the easy vocal onset behavior? It would be highly unlikely for a client to be able to follow instructions such as "As you start to exhale, bring the vocal folds together slowly." This is not normally a voluntary movement. And, even if the clinician models it, the client may not be able to produce the easy onset behavior. But if the clinician tells the client to say the word *hay* very slowly, she may indeed get the easy onset behavior to occur in the transition from the "h" to the "a" sound. The behavior is now a linguistic or phonemic movement rather than a purely motor function. It is a naturally occurring motor event in the word *hay*; it is reflexive, if you will. All of this is highly cognitive, both directly, with the client comprehending instructions and directions, and indirectly, in that the movement is part of the cognitively based phonology system.

Motor Learning

The term used most often in conjunction with motor learning is "perceptual-motor skills." The term is used to emphasize the relationship between sensory perception and the performance of the behavioral motor skill. This concept is often considered under the general heading of eye-hand coordination skills, such as holding a tennis racket or swinging a golf club. Although this may seem a bit abstract as applied to clients who have voice disorders, the principles involved in motor learning are of value in therapy. We might tend to view this as ear-larynx coordination. The major differences are that laryngeal movements cannot be observed as easily as hand movements and that the individual has less voluntary control over laryngeal movements than over hand movements.

Motor learning is complex and concerns the learning of a specific motor skill. A motor skill is most often taken to mean a chain or sequence of motor responses or muscular movements. They are learned through the coordination of various sensory and motor systems. The skill, once learned, is then incorporated into a larger response pattern. For example, a client may learn to change his pitch (a sequence of motor

—NOTES—

responses). He learned to do this by listening, watching and imitating, and once he had acquired the skill, he incorporated it into his speech, a larger response pattern. It is obvious that the primary sensory systems that are used in the application of motor learning are the visual and auditory systems.

There is a specific sequence involved in learning a new motor skill. The sequence involves the cognitive phase, the fixation phase, and finally the autonomous phase. In the first phase, the person doing the "teaching" provides information about the new behavior and models it. The person doing the "learning" then thinks about the information and the behavior, planning how he will attempt to perform it. When he has completed his planning, he then attempts the behavior. This process continues until the new behavior is relatively stable. The fixation phase consists of the learner practicing the new behavior until there are no errors in its performance. In the final phase, the autonomous phase, the learner speeds up and smooths out the performance to the point at which it is functional as a part of a larger unit of behavior.

In providing therapy for a client with a voice disorder, we follow the same sequence. In the cognitive phase we provide the client with information about the vocal behavior we want to teach and we also model it for him. The client thinks about this and plans how he will produce the behavior. He then attempts to reproduce the model as he perceived it. When reproduction is accurate, we move into the next phase of therapy, in which the behavior is practiced until there are no errors in production. The final phase of therapy consists of incorporating the new behavior into the client's on-going speech.

Behavioral Learning

We will now consider operant or instrumental conditioning. The most important thing to remember here is that the learning that occurs is dependent on the consequence of the behavior, that is, what happens after the behavior occurs. If the person views the consequence as positive, the behavior has been rewarded and the probability that it will occur again increases. However, if the person views the consequence as negative, there is a decreased probability of future occurrence of the behavior because it was penalized.

As can be seen, we learn either through rewards for our behaviors or through penalties for behaving in certain ways. If there is a reward each time we perform a behavior, we quickly learn to perform the behavior more often in order to get the reward. However, if the result of our performing a behavior is a penalty, we stop performing the behavior so that we can avoid the penalty.

Operant conditioning procedures are used in almost all therapy provided by speech clinicians. Some programs are reward oriented, whereas others are penalty oriented. But in the main, most clinical applications of these principles are combined so that the client receives both reward and penalty. Correct speech behaviors are encouraged to occur through rewards, whereas incorrect speech behaviors are discouraged through penalties.

When we use penalty we provide the client with negative "feedback" that indicates that the behavior he performed is not correct, not acceptable, or not performed as well as we know he can. We must respond to the client both positively and negatively in order to provide him with some guidance as he goes through the various steps of therapy.

Now, we need to extend this a bit further and understand that there are two forms of reward and two forms of penalty. The most common form of reward is to present the client with something he likes. If he likes chocolate, he is rewarded when he receives chocolate candy after performing a behavior. If he has learned the representative value of a token in a token economy (which will be discussed later), a token is also rewarding. This is a positive reward. We can also turn the concept around and remove a penalty that is in itself a reward, albeit a negative one. Owing to strict demands on the timing of this type of reward system it does not lend itself easily to a clinical situation. Therefore, we will forgo the clinical applications of this form of reward.

We had also mentioned that there are two forms of penalty. We can view them in the same way, the presenting of something negative or the removal of something positive. We penalize by application when we tell the client he did a poor job or when we make him repeat words he did not produce correctly. Penalty by removal would consist of taking away a toy he was playing with instead of attending to therapy, or removing a token if we are using a token economy.

ESTABLISHING A CLINICAL VOCABULARY

In order to discuss the treatment of vocal problems, we need to establish a clinical vocabulary. The following terms will be used throughout the book as we discuss therapy. The terminology that is unique to voice will be presented and discussed in later chapters.

Clinical Vocabulary

Behavior. A behavior is anything a person does. Overt behaviors are actions or movements that can be observed. Covert behaviors are thoughts, feelings, or motor performances that cannot be observed but are still behaviors. There is a concept known as the "dead man" rule that indicates that anything a living person can do that a "dead man" cannot do is a behavior. This should give us room to operate!

Behaviors have three characteristics that we will be concerned with: their frequency of occurrence, their strength or intensity when they occur, and their duration once they do occur. We will be manipulating these characteristics as we move through therapy.

Stimulus (S). A stimulus is anything that attracts a person's attention. It may be something inside the person such as a headache or something in his or her external environment, such as objects in a room. We will not view a stimulus as an event that "elicits" a behavior but rather as an event that prompts or cues a behavior to occur. The behavior may be either overt or covert.

Response (R). A response is the reaction a person has to a stimulus, a behavior. Responses would include thinking about the stimulus, looking at an object in a room, imitating a speech behavior presented by the clinician, rewarding a client for a correct behavior, and other such behaviors by either the client or the clinician.

Antecedent Event. An antecedent event is any event that precedes the response; that is, the stimulus that prompts or cues a response to occur.

Modeling. Modeling is the demonstration of a behavior. We show the clients what we want them to do. This could include such diverse behaviors as the producing of the [r] sound, speaking at a different pitch, opening the jaw farther during speech, slowing down the rate of speech, using the correct syntax, and so forth. These are demonstrations of the *behavior change goal* so that our clients know what we expect them to do.

Information. In our contact with the client we can either provide for the client or request from the client two types of information. First, we can provide *behavioral* information that is concerned with the behavior we are attempting to teach. This type of information might include telling the client to prolong the vowel when attempting to slow down the rate of speech or to open the mouth wider while speaking.

We can also request the client repeat what we have said to him to make sure he understood us.

Second, we can provide *general* information. This might include a description of our therapy, therapy goals, information to change attitudes or emotions, and so on. Again, we might ask the client to repeat what we have told him to determine his perception of what we said.

Guidance. Another term for guidance would be *prompt*. There are four types of guidance that we use in therapy. We give *verbal* guidance in the form of saying things that prompt the performance of a behavior. *Gestural* guidance would be those gestures used to prompt or cue a behavior to occur. We also use *environmental* guidance when we manipulate the environment so that it elicits the behavior, such as showing the client a picture. Finally, we use *physical* guidance when we actually touch the client to assist in the performance of a behavior.

Contingent Event. A contingent event is any event that follows the response. Basically, this means either a pleasant event (reward) or an unpleasant event (penalty).

Reward (R +). Reward means the same as reinforcement. A reward signifies a positive event that occurs after a behavior is performed. If the event is truly rewarding to the client, the chances of the behavior occurring again are increased.

Penalty (P). Penalty means the same as punishment. A penalty signifies a negative event that occurs after a behavior is performed. If the event is truly penalizing to the client, the chances of the behavior occurring again are decreased.

Extinguish. When reward for a behavior is withheld, the behavior will extinguish; that is, it will no longer occur since the reward is not presented and the behavior now has no purpose. However, if the behavior itself has become rewarding it will continue to occur since it is no longer dependent on an external reward.

Reward Schedule. When we use the term reward schedule, we refer to how often we reward a behavior. A *continuous schedule* means that we reward every occurrence of a behavior. This provides fast learning but the behavior is not very stable and will have a tendency to cease to occur when the reward is removed. With an *intermittent schedule* we reward on a more random basis. There are two types of intermittent systems, ratio and interval. In the ratio system, either fixed or variable, the reward is given based on the number of times the behavior has occurred. In the interval system, the determining factor for reward is time. The intermittent schedule is not as efficient for learning a behavior but makes the behavior very stable and the behavior will have a tendency to continue to occur even after the reward is removed.

Approach Motivation. Approach motivation represents the mental attitude of the client when the focus of therapy is on rewards. He will perform the behavior being rewarded more often in order to obtain more rewards.

Avoidance Motivation. Avoidance motivation represents the mental attitude of the client when the focus of therapy is on penalties. He will perform the behavior being penalized less often in order to avoid the penalty.

Shaping. Shaping is the process of creating a *new* behavior in a client. As behaviors more closely approximate the target behavior they are rewarded, and through this process the new behavior is gradually shaped.

Significant Others. Significant others are people who are very important in the client's life. They may be the client's parents, foster parents, relatives, wife, husband, close friends, or siblings.

Token Economy. When the client is initially rewarded with tokens, such as poker chips, that he can turn in at some later time for a more meaningful reward, this is referred to as a token economy.

Stimulus Control. Stimuli can be manipulated in several ways. They can be gradually presented, gradually withdrawn, increased in number, and decreased in number, or their prompting role can be changed.

Fading. Fading is the gradual removal of a stimulus. We can gradually withdraw our model of a behavior. We are then fading the model. Also, when we give the client a reward, it is a stimulus for him. When we gradually withdraw the rewards, we are fading them.

THE CLINICIAN/CLIENT INTERACTION

The clinical interactions between the clinician and the client are presented here as a series of "transactions." We will illustrate the transaction by using some of the terms just defined. The initial communication between the clinician and the client would appear as:

S — O — R

The (*S*) represents the clinician presenting the initial stimulus, the (*O*) stands for "organism" and represents the client's cognition of the stimulus; and the (*R*) represents the client's response to the clinician after he has thought about what he should do. It is now the clinician's turn to respond to the client. The diagram is then expanded to:

S—O—R/S—O—R

The (S) in this new part of the transaction now represents the client's response (R) as it becomes the stimulus (S) for the clinician. The (O) represents the clinician's cognition of the stimulus, and the (R) represents the clinician's response to the client. This completes the first transaction. In her cognitions during the transaction the clinician must (1) evaluate the correctness of the response for either a reward or a penalty, (2) determine if the correct response is occurring more often, (3) evaluate the attentiveness of the client to the therapy, and (4) determine how to initiate the next transaction. The direction of the next transaction is dependent on how successful the current transaction has been. If the client's response was correct and the client was attending to therapy, she can proceed to the next step in therapy. If the response was not correct or the client was not attending to therapy, she will have to repeat this transaction or deal with the client's lack of attentiveness.

The kind of response the clinician gives to the client is extremely important. If the response is a reward, she will be creating approach motivation in the client. However, if the response is a penalty, she will be creating avoidance motivation in the client. These forms of motivation are vital to successful therapy and are directly controlled by the clinician. Both motivational forms will be used in our therapy so it is important that you recognize their basic differences. With approach motivation the client is actively seeking the reward, whereas with avoidance motivation the client is actively seeking to avoid the penalty.

There are *two* behavioral performances occurring in each transaction: the clinical behavior that the clinician is focusing on and the attending behavior of the client. Rewards and penalties will influence both forms of behavior. If attending behavior is rewarded, it will occur more often and, conversely, nonattending behavior will occur less often when it is penalized. Because the client must be attending to therapy if it is to be effective, the focus of therapy may occasionally shift to dealing with attending behaviors.

Having completed the first transaction, the clinician initiates the second transaction. This sequence then continues, with the direction of each transaction dependent on the preceding one. If you will, the

—NOTES—

transactions are like a string of beads—the clinician adds each bead to the string after the preceding one is in place. Another way to view the clinical transaction is in a circular mode, as shown in Figure 1.

Each time the circle is completed it represents a clinical transaction. Consider the following example of two transactions with a voice client:

S—Clinician demonstrates (models) easy vocal onset.
O—Client perceives and thinks about the model.
R—Client initiates voice, attempting to imitate the model.
S—Client's vocal onset is the stimulus for the clinician.
O—Clinician evaluates the client's vocal behavior.
R—Clinician says, "That was a little hard. Let's try it again" (penalty).
(End first transaction)
S—Clinician models easy vocal onset again.
O—Client perceives and thinks about the model.
R—Client initiates voice, attempting to imitate the model.

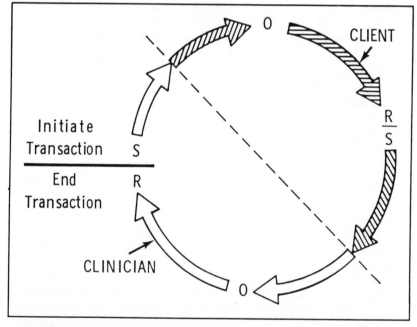

FIGURE 1
Clinical Transaction Diagram. The clinical transaction is initiated by the clinician's stimulus (S). The client thinks about the stimulus (O) and then responds (R). The client's response is the stimulus (S) for the clinician. She evaluates the client's stimulus (O) and then responds (R). This constitutes one clinical transaction. The clinician's next stimulus (S) initiates the next transaction.

S—Client's vocal onset is the stimulus for the clinician.

O—Clinician evaluates the client's vocal behavior.

R—Clinician says, "That was very good, just like I did it" (reward).

(End second transaction)

Transactional Testing

Each transaction represents the clinician's testing of how well the client is learning, the effectiveness of the rewards and penalties, and his attending to therapy. This testing is basic to therapy. It determines if a transaction must be repeated, if the focus of therapy must be shifted to attending behaviors, if the reward or the penalty must be changed, and how effective and efficient the therapy is. One of the most important aspects of testing concerns the effects the clinician's responses are having on the client, in terms of both the speech behavior and the attending behaviors. It is very important for the clinician to respond in some way to the client after each of his responses. The clinician may actually extinguish a new behavior by not responding to it. A behavior must have a reason to be performed, namely, a reward of some kind.

THE CLINICIAN'S TASKS

As was indicated in the transactional diagram, the clinician has three specific tasks in each transaction. She must first provide the stimulus to start the transaction and prompt the client's response. Her next task is to evaluate the client's response and, finally, to respond to the client.

The Clinician's Stimulus (Starting the Transaction)

Modeling. Perhaps the most common form of stimulus used by the speech clinician is to "model" the behavior for the client. When we speak of modeling, we are talking about the clinician demonstrating the behavior so that the client can attempt to imitate it. We are setting forth the behavior change goal for the client with the model. When he sees or hears the model he knows what the clinician expects him to do. With voice clients it is doubly important that we recognize that there are both auditory and visual aspects of the model. The behaviors we will be modeling have very little visual impact, since most vocal behaviors cannot be directly seen. Therefore, the model is primarily an auditory one.

—NOTES—

Guidance. Guidance is leading or directing the client to the correct behavior or prompting it to occur. It can take the form of verbal, gestural, environmental, or physical guidance. An example of verbal guidance would be to say to a client, "Speak a bit lower; you are talking too high." Verbal guidance (or verbal prompts) assist in the production of a behavior when the model is not present. Facial expressions and body or hand gestures are part of gestural guidance. Again, these are used to prompt a behavior to occur or to modify it. If we gesture in such a way to indicate that the client speak louder, this would be gestural guidance. When we manipulate or change the clinical environment so that a desired behavior occurs, this is environmental guidance. An example of environmental guidance would be to take a client whose vocal problem is due to tension and put him in a relaxing chair. With increased relaxation, there would be less vocal deviation. If we assist the relaxation by massaging the neck muscles of the client, we add physical guidance. The various forms of guidance can be used in any combination.

Information. There are two types of information. Behavioral information is information we give the client about how to produce the behavior he is attempting to perform. We might tell the client that when he attempts to use easy vocal onset, he should start speaking by using a very short [h] sound which will create easy onset. General information is that information we give our client that is related to therapy but not to the specific behavior. This would constitute such information as telling him when the next therapy session will be or giving him work to do at home.

We can also ask the client for information, for instance, asking him if he understands what we are telling him. We might have him repeat what we have said to see if he is paying attention. Other information we might want from some vocal clients would concern their feelings about their voice problem. We should do this as we are doing the initial evaluation of the voice.

The Clinician's Cognitions

The clinician must make some very important decisions after she hears or sees the client's response. She is involved in evaluating the correctness of the response, determining if the correct response is occurring more often, evaluating the client's attentiveness to therapy, and deciding how she will start the next transaction.

The first three decisions determine if she moves ahead in therapy or if she must repeat the last transaction. This testing also tells her if she must shift her therapy from focusing on the speech to dealing with the client's attending behaviors and his approach or avoidance motivation.

With some voice clients, the clinician must also be aware of the client's cognitive set: his attitudes, emotions, and feelings during the transactions. If any of these factors begin to negatively influence the treatment program, the clinician must deal with them. If these factors are positively influencing treatment, the clinician should take advantage of the opportunity to reward the positive cognitive set. In some instances in which the negative influence is totally disrupting treatment, the focus of therapy may have to be shifted for a period of time while the clinician deals with the client's cognitions through counseling.

The Clinician's Responses (Ending the Transaction)

Reward. The reward is an event that occurs following the behavior, an event that the client sees as a positive consequence. Through approach motivation, the client is motivated to get the reward by performing a behavior that will be rewarded. Approach motivation is extremely important to therapy. However, in selecting something for a reward, we must remember that we can not determine if it is actually a reward until its effect on the client's behavior is studied. An event can only be labeled a "reward" if its presentation results in an increase in the frequency of occurrence of the behavior. Many clinicians decide on a "reward" by selecting things THEY feel are rewarding but never check to see what effect it is having on the client and his behavior. You may feel that a very chewy candy is a reward, but if the client has braces on his teeth, this could be a penalty for the client. However, if therapy must wait until the candy is cleaned from the braces and your therapy is boring, the delay, not the candy, may be the reward for the client. Rewards must be selected with the client's likes and dislikes in mind. So, when we make a decision on what we are going to use as a reward, we must observe the effect that it has on the client and the behavior.

The two types of rewards we can give our clients are primary rewards and secondary rewards. Primary rewards are directed to basic needs such as food and water. Secondary rewards are more social in nature and are learned. These would include examples such as verbally praising the client or giving the client a token as a reward. With either form of reward we must consider the strength and the timing of the reward, how appropriate it is for our clinical setting, and how often we present it.

The strength of the reward is dependent on how important it is to the client. If the reward is of little value to the client, it is not a strong reward. However, if the reward is highly valued by the client, it is a strong reward. The stronger the reward, the higher the client's approach motivation; he will be highly motivated to get the reward. Further, if the clinician has a good rapport with the client, any reward is strengthened because the clinician is an important person to the client, and this makes the reward more significant.

The timing of the reward is crucial. There cannot be too long a period of time between the performance of the behavior and the receiving of the reward. The client must associate the performance of the specific behavior with the presentation of the reward. If another behavior occurs between the desired behavior and the presentation of the reward, it is the second behavior that is being rewarded since the reward is contingent to it.

The appropriateness of the reward must also be considered. Food is not an appropriate reward if the client is to consume it immediately after it is presented; as with our example of the chewy candy, this may take up the rest of the time scheduled for therapy. It would be better if the client had to wait until after therapy to consume it. The client would now have to get the candy out of his braces on his own time, not during clinical time. More appropriate rewards would be verbal praise, stickers (stars, characters, science fiction), an ink stamp on the hand, additional recess or library time, transfers, plastic toys, or tokens.

The schedule of presentation of the reward must also be considered. The two types of reward schedules are *continuous* and *intermittent*. With the continuous reward schedule, the reward is presented every time the behavior is performed, in other words, in a ratio of 1 to 1. This leads to rapid learning but also, when the reward is removed, rapid extinction; that is, the behavior disappears quickly when the reward is removed.

With the intermittent reward schedule we no longer reward every behavioral performance. We may reward every other performance (a 2 to 1 ratio) or every third performance (a 3 to 1 ratio). We can also reward more on a random basis. This type of schedule does not lend itself to rapid learning, but it does reduce the effect of extinction. The behavior tends to continue even after the reward has been removed since there is still a chance that a reward will be forthcoming. In therapy, we normally start out with a continuous reward schedule for fast learning and then shift to an intermittent schedule to resist extinction when the rewards are eliminated.

There are some people who object to the use of rewards in therapy. They feel that the client is being bribed to perform their new speech behavior, and the word *bribe* has negative connotations. If the reward is viewed as "payment" for work done, then the concept of a bribe is avoided. This also gives us a means of explaining our clinical procedure to parents who might object to rewards from this standpoint. This can be explained to a working parent by drawing an analogy between receiving a paycheck for work he or she has accomplished and the reward the child receives for clinical "work" he has accomplished.

Penalty. Theoretically, if the incorrect productions of a speech behavior are ignored, that is, if there is no contingent event, the behavior should extinguish. However, the incorrect speech behavior is usually strongly habituated and self-rewarding. A more efficient means of dealing with incorrect speech productions is to penalize their occurrence in some way. Most clinicians respond to incorrect productions by saying to the client, "That was not very good" or "I think you can do that better." This is a form of penalty. Penalty does not have to be harsh or severe. When the client is informed that the production was not correct, if this is interpreted by the client as a penalty, there will be a decrease in occurrence of the incorrect behavior. The client will develop avoidance motivation and will not perform the behavior that is penalized. Penalizing the behavior is a more efficient way to eliminate a behavior than relying on extinction to occur.

We must apply the same rules to a penalty that we applied to a reward. We must determine if our response is actually a penalty, determine the strength of the penalty, consider the contingency (or timing) of the penalty, and consider the appropriateness of the penalty. A response can be considered a penalty only if the frequency of occurrence of the penalized behavior decreases. The strength of the penalty must also be carefully considered as well as how often it is applied. As was stated earlier, the penalty need not be severe or harsh, just strong enough so that the client would prefer to avoid it. We must be careful not to apply too many penalties, since this has a negative effect on the morale of the client, and when we apply a penalty, we should also be consistent in its application. Nothing is more disconcerting than to be penalized inconsistently for something. Finally, we must decide on a penalty that is appropriate not only for the client but also for the work environment. A clinician who levies a fine of one dollar for each occurrence of an incorrect response might perhaps make a lot of money early in therapy but would sooner or later face some problems with her administration. Public institutions such as the schools are sensitive to public opinion, and the penalty you use should be carefully determined.

—NOTES—

The two basic forms of penalty are penalty by administration and by withdrawal. We can administer such penalties as requiring the client to repeat a behavior or giving him verbal penalty. Penalty by withdrawal would constitute the removal of a reward, such as the removal of a token or a distracting object. We can also remove the client from the clinical environment where he receives rewards. This does not necessarily mean having the client leave therapy and return to the classroom. With some therapy the authors have observed, this would be a reward for the client. If the client is in a group in which he is receiving rewards and we remove him from the group, we have removed his opportunity to receive rewards. This is a form of "time out" and is a commonly used form of penalty. However, with either form of penalty we are still creating avoidance motivation, as the client attempts to avoid the penalty by not performing the behavior.

Again, we will find people who object to the use of penalty with a client. The use of penalty in therapy creates more negative reactions than the use of reward. However, if we think carefully about all learning environments, penalty is a common feature. All parents use some form of penalty in raising their children. There are obvious exceptions in which parents never penalize their children, regardless of their behavior and most clinicians have a special name for these children. But we must also recognize that all speech clinicians use some form of penalty in their therapy, even if no more than telling the client that he did not perform the behavior correctly. All people learn to avoid things through penalty. It is a valuable form of learning.

THE CLINICAL INTERACTION MODEL

We will now combine the learning orientations with the clinician-client transactions to form a model of clinical interactions. The Clinical Interaction Model (CIM) is presented in Figure 2. The basic (S—O—R/S—O—R) transaction has been expanded in this model to include all the clinician's and client's activities. It also illustrates the influence of the clinician's responses, either reward or penalty, on the client's approach and avoidance motivations and his attending behaviors. This model will serve as a clinical guide for voice therapy. The CIM will also be of assistance in analyzing any problems you might have in therapy, such as the client not comprehending your model or information. The key word associated with both the clinician's stimulus and her response is "appropriate." The judgment of appropriateness is a clinical judgment that only the clinician can make, but she should be aware that if adjustment must be made in therapy, the adjustment should be made by the clinician in terms of her modifying her stimulus, her response, or both. For example, if the clinician presents the client with information that is too complex, that is, beyond the cognitive level of the client, constant repetition of the information will accomplish nothing except to frustrate the client. In order to have the client comprehend the information, the clinician must adjust it to the cognitive level of the client. This might mean rephrasing the information or changing the terminology used. Further, if the clinician is requesting a behavioral performance that is beyond the ability of the client, she again creates frustration in the client. The clinician must recognize that her behavioral request was not appropriate for the functional level of the client. The stimulus from the clinician must be appropriate for the individual client.

The concept of "appropriateness" also applies to the clinician's rewards and penalties. As was stated earlier, they must be appropriate for the client and for the work environment, *and the client is the only one who can determine if the clinician's response is a reward or a penalty* . A reward or penalty is not appropriate if the client does not interpret it as such. There are also rewards and penalties that are not appropriate for various clinical environments. The clinician must make this judgment as she assesses her work environment.

Finally, the CIM also demonstrates the relationship between the speech (voice) behavior and the attending behavior of the client. Appropriate rewards and penalties will maintain the client's approach and avoidance motivations and this fosters the attending behavior. However, if the client loses his motivation he will not be attending to therapy. In this instance the clinician must shift her clinical focus from the speech behavior to attending behavior, because the client will not learn if he is not paying attention. The clinician must re-evaluate her reward and penalty and modify them if they have lost their effect. Having done this, she could reward the client's attending behavior or penalize the nonattending behavior as she tells a story. She will have temporarily shifted therapy from the speech behavior to attending behavior. However, once the client's attention and motivation are re-established, she can shift back to the speech behavior, making sure she does not lose the client's attention as she does so. This is a vital aspect of the CIM, since all therapy is dependent on the client's attending to the clinician.

Before we leave the discussion of the CIM, let us go through the model step by step. The clinical interaction begins with the clinician's stimulus, which is a combination of the factors listed in the CIM. The next step is the client's cognition, or thinking about the stimulus. After

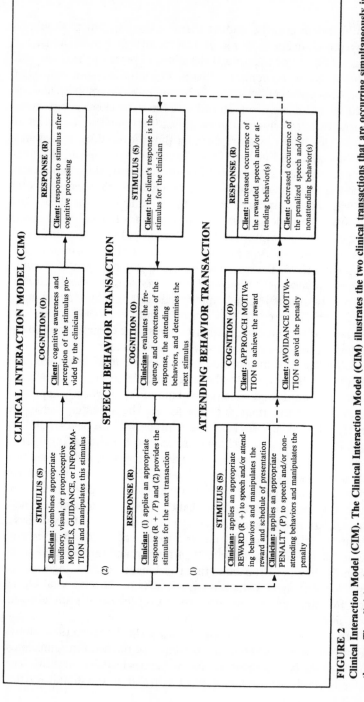

FIGURE 2

Clinical Interaction Model (CIM). The Clinical Interaction Model (CIM) illustrates the two clinical transactions that are occurring simultaneously in therapy. The clinician is attending to the speech behaviors of the client as well as to his attending behaviors. The focal point of therapy is the speech behavior, but if the attending behavior becomes a problem, she can focus her therapy of the client's motivation and attending behaviors. Her response to the client, either reward or penalty, is very critical. It not only affects the occurrences of the client's speech behaviors but also influences the client's motivation in therapy.

thinking about the stimulus the client responds. This response is the stimulus for the clinician, and she then thinks about and evaluates the response in terms of the frequency and correctness of the response, the client's attention to therapy, and how to start the next transaction. When her evaluation is completed, she responds to the client with either a reward or a penalty. The next transaction is now ready to begin. However, the clinician's reward or penalty also has an effect on the client's attending behaviors, his motivation. Rewards increase the approach motivation, whereas penalties increase the avoidance motivation. These then have the effect of increasing the occurrences of attending behaviors and the speech behavior (rewards) or decreasing the occurrences of non-attending behaviors or the incorrect speech behavior (penalties). During therapy the clinician focuses on the speech behavior transactions while monitoring the client's motivation and attending behavior. If a problem with motivation and attention exists, she shifts her focus to these areas until she again has the client's attention and motivation. She can then shift therapy back to the speech behaviors.

The CIM represents *all* of your clinical interactions. It applies not only to your client but to all interaction when you are attempting to teach a new concept, belief, or behavior or when you are gathering information, such as during an interview or an evaluation. You will use the CIM in a teaching mode with your client, his parents, and his teacher. If you have a home program for a client you will have to teach the parents how to carry on the program. You will also teach the classroom teacher how to respond to the client if you involve her in the program. The information-gathering mode will also be used with the client, the parents, and the teacher as you monitor your program's success in the home and other talking environments. The CIM is the core of all clinical transactions.

STIMULUS CONTROL

Before we leave this chapter on therapy, we need to consider one other important principle that will influence our therapy. This has to do with *stimulus control*, the manipulation of stimuli in order to influence the performance of behavior. This is an important feature in all phases of therapy, but especially important when we generalize the new vocal behaviors to other environments. Thus far discussion of the stimulus has been limited to that which is provided by the clinician. We will now broaden our view to include other forms of stimuli which influence the client.

—NOTES—

Conditioned Stimuli

Stimuli that are consistently associated with reward or penalty become conditioned so that they "cue" the client as to what the outcome will be if a particular behavior is performed. Conditioned stimuli are referred to as *discriminative stimuli*. They do not *elicit* a behavioral response, but rather prompt or cue the behavior to occur or to be avoided. Because the individual knows what the outcome will be if he performs the behavior, he has some influence over whether or not the behavior occurs. Positive cues will encourage the performance of a response while negative cues will discourage the performance of a response. Thus, the stimulus cues have a direct influence on the probability of the behavior occurring.

Positive Stimuli. Stimuli which have been conditioned to a positive outcome—a reward—will be referred to as *positive stimuli*, or $S+$. A glass of iced tea on a hot day has become an $S+$ to many of us. The tea signifies that if we drink it, the outcome will be rewarding. The iced tea was not originally a conditioned stimulus. It became conditioned $S+$ only after we had drunk some on a hot day and found it rewarding: An association was then made between the iced tea and the reward of drinking it.

In that rewards are associated with therapy, stimuli in that environment quickly assume the role of $S+$. When a speech behavior is rewarded and the reward is associted with the clinician, she becomes an $S+$. Thus, when the clinician is present, the client is cued that if the specific speech behavior is performed, he will be rewarded. Even the clinic room becomes an $S+$ role, cuing the behavior that is rewarded to occur.

Negative Stimuli. Stimuli associated with a negative outcome, a penalty, assume the role of a negative stimuli, or $S-$. There are many such cues in our lives. $S-$ cues, for example, influence the way we drive our cars. Let us say that we are driving our car a bit over the posted speed limit when police car, an $S-$, is sighted. We quickly reduce our speed to the posted limit so as to avoid receiving a speeding ticket, a rather severe penalty. We know that driving too fast results in a traffic ticket, so we avoid the ticket by not performing the behavior. (What happens to the speed of our car when the patrol car is out of sight is left to your imagination.)

Signs often serve as $S-$ cues. This would include signs such as *Keep Out, Do Not Enter, Beware of the Dog, Wrong Way, Do Not Touch,* and *If It Breaks, You Bought It.* Doors with the signs *Men* or

Women on them can also assume an S− role, especially when we have just entered the wrong one.

If the client performs a behavior and the clinician responds by penalizing him, she assumes the role of S− for that behavior. The behavior may be a disruptive behavior such as wandering around the clinic room, nonattending behavior in the form of looking out the window, or an incorrect speech behavior. The S− role is important not only in direct therapy, but also in establishing control over clients whose behaviors interfere with therapy.

If the client avoids the penalty by not performing the negative behavior, what behavior does he perform? He will search for a behavior that will not be penalized, or if the clinician has taught him an alternate behavior he will perform it, especially when it results in a reward. By performing the behavior the clinician has taught him, he can not only avoid the penalty but also achieve the reward. For example, a client is talking to the clinician and his pitch goes up. He immediately senses that he will be penalized by the clinician (S−) for the high pitch; he additionally recognizes the clinician as an S+ for a lower pitch and shifts to a lower pitch. By doing this he not only avoids the penalty (a form of negative reward) but also gets a direct reward. Thus, the lower pitch is rewarded twice.

Neutral Stimuli. In addition to the stimulus roles of S+ (prompting the correct production of the speech behavior) and S− (prompting the avoidance of the penalty by not producing the incorrect behavior) the clinican can assume a third stimulus role. This is the role of a neutral stimulus, or *S0*. This stimulus cues that there will be no consequence for a given behavior. If a behavior is not rewarded (or rewarding), it has no purpose, no reason to exist, and the behavior extinguishes.

Stimulus Manipulation

The clinician is able to manipulate these stimuli in a number of ways. The five forms of stimulus manipulation are very important to therapy and will be discussed individually.

Shifting the role of the Stimuli. A stimulus may have been conditioned to an S+, S−, or S0 role, but these roles can be changed. If the client's parents have been penalizing him for his high pitch, their role is an S−. However, if they are counseled so that they no longer penalize the client's pitch, their role will shift to S0. If the parents have been rewarding the high pitch in the home, their role is an S+. Their

—NOTES—

S + role can be shifted to an S0 by removing the reward. The stimulus role can be changed by associating the stimulus with a different contingent event. This will be an important factor in establishing a home program to supplement clinical work. This is especially important when the new speech is generalized to environments outside the clinic room.

A rule of thumb in shifting stimulus roles is that any stimulus, regardless of its current role, becomes an S + when consistently associated with reward. When associated with penalty, stimuli become S −, and when there is no contingent event they become S0.

Gradual Introduction of Stimuli. An S − that is too threatening and overwhelms the client must be introduced gradually, allowing the client time to adjust to it. A client may find it extremely frightening to speak in front of a group. When he is in front of a group, he is so frightened and tense that he can not use his new speaking pitch. We can gradually introduce this S − situation by starting with one listener. When the client can perform satisfactorily with one listener and the situation becomes an S + , another listener can be added. This process is repeated. We are gradually introducing the stimuli, while keeping the situation at an emotional level at which the client can perform his new speech behavior. The speaking situation gradually then shifts from an S − to an S + (or at least a very weak S −) as he learns that he can speak in front of a group. In this example we are gradually increasing the strength or intensity of the stimulus. We can also manipulate the frequency and duration of a stimuli if and when the need arises.

Gradual Withdrawal of Stimuli. The stimulus can also be gradually withdrawn or faded. We do this by presenting it less often (*frequency*), in a weaker form (*strength* or *intensity*), or for an shorter period of time (*duration*). We can fade the model as the client learns the new speech behavior, or we can fade the influence of our S + role by not rewarding as much. Fading makes the new speech behavior more independent. We must eventually fade all stimuli so that the new speech behavior is being performed independently of prompts or cues. When this is happening, we can terminate therapy.

Increase the Number of Stimuli. We must increase the number of S + in the client's speaking environments if we are to achieve carryover of the new speech behavior. These S + will cue the new speech behavior to occur in other environments, such as in the school, the home, and on the job. This form of manipulation is dependent on the client's significant others or cooperative people in those environments. This form of stimulus manipulation is extrememly important. The efficiency of therapy in terms of generalizing the new speech to other speaking environments is dependent upon the number of S+ in the client's life.

Decrease the Number of Stimuli. We may need to reduce the number of stimuli in the client's clinical environment. The client may be overwhelmed by the number of other clients in a group or other distractions in the clinical room. If the client cannot function in a large group, he may be placed in a smaller group or even given individual therapy until he can handle a small group (gradual introduction of stimuli). If he is distressed by an object in the room, it may be removed. To many clients, a tape recorder is an S−, and its presence may interfere with therapy.

We can now conclude our discussion of the principles of cognitive behavior therapy and other factors which influence our clinical interactions with our clients. The answers to the word puzzles earlier in the chapter? See if you recognized the following: (1) break in pitch, (2) vocal intensity, and (3) subglottal air pressure.

Chapter 3

Vocal Mechanics

INTRODUCTION

It was stressed earlier that the effectiveness and efficiency of your therapy would be dependent on how well you understood the operation of the vocal system. This chapter is a brief review of the process of vocal production, and, yes, there will be some anatomy and physiology involved but we will try to keep it to a minimum. Let us begin by defining some of the basic terms we will be using. We will start with the term *vocal mechanics,* because it is the chapter title and might need some clarification:

Vocal Mechanics. Vocal mechanics is the study of forces operating on the larynx to produce adjustments and vibrations necessary for speech. The factors involved in these adjustments are the anatomy and physiology of the larynx and the principles of aerodynamics.

Anatomy. Anatomy is the study of the structure (architecture) of an organism like the human body.

Physiology. Physiology is the study of the functions of the anatomy.

Aerodynamics. Aerodynamics is the study of air motion and air flow.

Let us consider an example of vocal behavior and see how our terms apply. Speech production, including voice, is the end product of an air driven system. Our study of anatomy, physiology, mechanics, and aerodynamics is useful only in that we can describe and understand what happens to the air stream as it is influenced by these factors. For example, when the lateral cricoarytenoid muscles contract, the vocal folds approximate (come together). As they approximate, air escaping from the lungs by way of the trachea sets them into vibration. The result of this vibration is that the air stream is divided into individual puffs of air rather than a continuous flow. The number of puffs of air per unit time gives the voice pitch. The vigor with which these puffs are released is associated with air pressure and gives the voice loudness. Now, let us apply our definitions to this example.

Vocal Mechanics: Adduction (bringing together) of the vocal folds, plus impeding or partially blocking the outward flow of air
Anatomy: Lateral cricoarytenoid muscles, arytenoid cartilages, vocal folds
Physiology: Rotation of the arytenoid cartilages laterally; movement of the vocal folds medially
Aerodynamics: The breaking up of a continuous air stream into puffs of air that constitute the vocal tone

The production of voice is dependent on three related physiological and acoustic events. First, respiration must provide an outward flow of air in order for there to be breath support for the voice. Second, the larynx must provide phonation, the modification of the flow of air into the individual puffs of air. Finally, the vocal tone is modified by the resonators in the vocal tract to give the vocal tone individualistic identity. We will discuss each of these physiological or acoustic events and then tie them all together, showing how, in concert, they produce voice.

RESPIRATION

Respiration for speech production is usually thought of as the source of power for the system. Of particular interest to us is how the respiratory system, normally used for oxygenation of the blood (gas exchange), is modified to supply the power for speech. We need to understand how the power is provided, how much power is needed, how to determine when the system is not performing satisfactorily, and what effect this has on voice production. The most basic structures involved here are the lungs.

The lungs are housed inside of the thorax (rib cage). The rib cage provides two very important functions. First, by the nature of its design, the rib cage provides protection for the lungs and the heart. Second, because of the way in which the lungs attach to the ribs, the lungs follow the movements of the rib cage faithfully. On the inner side of the rib cage and on the outer side of the lungs, there is a strong protective covering, or sheathing material. In between these two coverings is an oily substance called synovial fluid. It is this oily fluid that sticks the two together, much like wetting two pieces of paper and sticking them together. Thus, as the rib cage moves, so do the lungs.

The anatomical and physiological importance of the lung–rib cage unity is that several muscles that attach to the rib cage can expand it. When the rib cage is expanded, the lungs expand and create a negative air pressure inside them. Then, according to a law of physics, air from outside rushes in to fill the new space and to equalize the pressure. This is called inhalation. If we now decrease the size of the rib cage and the lungs, the reverse happens; this is exhalation.

Breathing for speech is a unique form of respiration. Normal exhalation requires no muscle activity. Normal forces such as tissue elasticity and the torque of the twisted ribs restore the lungs to the rest position, reduce the size of the lungs, and expel air (exhalation). Since we speak on exhaled air, the role of respiration for speech is to control the natural forces of exhalation. The process of controlling the rapid exhalation of air to provide a constant flow of air and to lengthen the time necessary to talk is the result of using the muscles of inhalation against the forces of exhalation. Thus, it is important that we first understand the inhalation process both for getting air in and for holding back rapid exhalation.

The most important muscle of inhalation for speech is the diaphragm. This bowl-shaped muscle separates the rib cage from the abdomen. When the diaphragm contracts, it tends to flatten and in doing so lowers the floor of the rib cage (thorax), pushing the viscera down; as the abdomen extends out, this vertical expansion of the thorax increases its dimensions, which increases the dimensions of the lungs. Air rushes in to fill the new space. The diaphragm clearly is the single most important muscle of inhalation because of its ability to increase the size of the thorax.

Simultaneous with the contraction of the diaphragm, other muscles whose function is to elevate the rib cage come into play. As the diaphragm is lowering the floor of the thorax, other muscles are elevating the rib cage and, because of the unique design of the ribs, increasing its horizontal dimensions. As the area within the rib cage is expanded, both vertically and horizontally, the lungs are also expanded and we inhale. Exhalation begins immediately after the inhalation phase is completed. As the rib cage is lowered, the diaphragm is returned to the rest position by way of natural forces. If we wish to contract the abdominal muscles, we can force the diaphragm back to the rest position. Contraction of the abdominal muscles will result in a forced exhalation, which is unnecessary for normal speech production but often found in professional uses of the voice.

Even though the respiratory cycle is now adequate to set the vocal folds into vibration, we must recognize that an unmodified exhalation is not appropriate for speech production. First, a 1 or 2 second exhalation is not enough time for most utterances. Second, we need to control the release of air so that the air pressure at the end of exhalation is equal to the air pressure at the beginning of exhalation. If air pressure is not controlled, the voice may vary in loudness as well as create potential problems for the precision required for speech articulation. Uncontrolled air pressure may also set the vocal folds into a violent initiation of phonation, possibly leading to vocal abuse and pathologic changes in the vocal apparatus.

The very important process of equalizing air pressure throughout an exhalation for speech production is known as *checking action*. By definition, checking action involves the muscles of inhalation working during exhalation to control and regulate the pressure and volume of air flow. In addition to the diaphragm muscle, the muscles found between the ribs, the intercostals, appear to be active during checking action. In reality, any muscle found in the thoracic region is potentially a muscle of inhalation (because it can increase the size of the rib cage) and is therefore also a potential muscle for checking the exhalation.

We cannot overemphasize the importance of checking action in speech production. Although disagreement continues to exist as to why and how checking action takes place, we must acknowledge that this is an extremely important behavior in normal voice production. A speaker may have excellent control over his laryngeal system and vocal behaviors, but if his respiratory system is providing an inconsistent air flow, abnormal vocal behaviors will occur.

PHONATION

Physics of Vibration

We would like to begin this aspect of vocal mechanics with a statement about vibration. For all practical purpose, everything physical in the universe vibrates. The chair you are sitting on is vibrating, as is every piece of furniture in the room. Skyscrapers vibrate, as does the car you drive. There are, however, two types of vibration, natural and forced. When things vibrate naturally, they tend to establish their own natural frequency and intensity based on their length, tension, and mass. Objects can also be forced to vibrate. If we set a tuning fork on a table, the table will begin to vibrate at the frequency of the tuning fork. If the tuning fork and the table naturally vibrate at about the same frequency or multiples of the frequency, then they are said to be in harmony. If, however, the tuning fork vibrates at a different frequency than the table, then the table is "forced" to vibrate at the frequency of the tuning fork. This forced vibration, if allowed to persist and if intense enough, will result in the table coming apart. Thus, the general notion that forced vibration has negative effects on an object is a very important concept to remember.

The basic concept here is that all objects have a natural period of vibration but that they can also be forced to vibrate at another frequency. The vocal folds also have a natural period of vibration based on their length, tension, and mass but they too can be forced to vibrate at another frequency. Vocal folds that are forced to vibrate at an unnatural frequency may suffer from vocal abuse, forming vocal nodules or showing other forms of tissue change.

Earlier we concluded that the major responsibility of the respiratory system was to provide a constant air flow or energy source and to check the flow of air to regulate its pressure over time. When the vocal folds are approximated and vibrating, they are also involved in the overall checking action, regulating the amount of air that is allowed to escape from the lungs. Thus, if the vocal folds cannot properly approximate, this has an adverse influence on the checking action. However, in the context of our discussion of vocal mechanics, we will assume that proper vocal fold approximation exists.

Vocal Fold Vibration

The vocal folds in concert with the entire laryngeal system are responsible for three distinct functions: producing voice or voicing (as opposed to voiceless exhalation, or "unvoicing," if you will), raising and lowering the vocal pitch, and increasing and decreasing the vocal loudness. Each of these functions are normally managed by the intrinsic muscles of the larynx. It is important to note that each function can be performed independently; that is, we can change pitch and leave loudness and voicing unchanged, or we can change loudness and not change pitch and voicing. Of course, when we stop voicing there is no longer pitch or loudness, but the point is that the independence of these major functions should indicate to us that there are separate muscles that are responsible for each function. This is a controversial issue, especially in regard to trained singers, but we are interested in clients whose voices are substandard or deviant so we will assume this stand for sake of our therapy.

Voice. If we close the space between the vocal folds (glottis) gently, the vocal folds will begin to vibrate freely and naturally at a point or distance that is just short of actually touching. This vocal fold approximation is accomplished by the lateral cricoarytenoid muscle. Because this adduction is accomplished by the rotation of the arytenoid cartilages and due to the posterior attachment of the vocal folds, this type of adduction takes more time than adduction for biological purposes (such as coughing). (You can get a sense of the time requirements if you slowly exhale, gradually introduce phonation, then return to a constant air flow, then return to vocalizing, and so on). If only the lateral cricoarytenoid muscle is providing adduction, a glottal or hard vocal attack is impossible. However, if another muscle normally involved in the biological adduction of the folds is also used, you will hear a hard glottal attack and the air stream will be interrupted between phonations.

The posterior cricoarytenoid muscles separate or open the vocal folds and create an open airway, or a glottis, between them. These two muscles clearly have the responsibility of gentle adduction for voicing and gentle abduction for unvoicing.

Pitch. The frequency of natural vibration of the vocal folds is dependent on their length, tension, and mass. If we wish to change the vibrating frequency of the vocal folds, we need only to change these components. Stringed instruments use the identical factors. Change the length, tension, or mass of the string and you change its pitch. When we play a stringed instrument, we change only one of these factors. However, when we "play" the vocal folds, we change all of the factors and all at the same time. It is much like a rubber band. Stretch it out, pluck it, and it vibrates. Stretch it out further and the pitch (frequency) goes up. We have increased its length and tension while decreasing its mass. In the same way, if we lengthen the vocal folds, we also increase their tension and decrease their mass. The end result is that the pitch goes up. If we shorten the vocal folds, the tension lessens and the mass increases and the pitch comes down. There are two sets of muscles involved in these adjustments for pitch, the cricothyroids and the thyroarytenoids.

Although there is some controversy regarding the actions of the cricothyroids and the thyroarytenoids in changing pitch, we are assuming the position that when the cricothyroids contract they pull the thyroid cartilage down and slide it forward. The result of this action is that the vocal folds are lengthened. When the thyroarytenoids contract they pull the thyroid cartilage up and slide it back, shortening the vocal folds. Even though the thyroarytenoid muscles are themselves the vocal folds, they work in conjunction with the cricothyroid muscles to control pitch. The muscles work in concert to maintain the appropriate length, tension, and mass to produce the desired vocal pitch. For further information on the interactions between the cricothyroid and thyroarytenoid muscles, the reader is referred to the readings listed in the References and Recommended Readings section.

Loudness. The concept of loudness is somewhat more complex. A common belief is that if the air stream is "pushed out harder," increasing subglottal air pressure, the voice will automatically be louder. Although there is some truth in this concept, the vocal mechanism is capable of producing the necessary range of loudness needed for normal speech production with minimal changes in subglottal air pressure. This laryngeal control of loudness allows the respiratory system to concentrate on providing a constant flow of air. If we involved respiration in subtle changes of loudness, we would upset the aerodynamic properties of the vocal system.

How does the larynx increase the loudness of the voice? The interarytenoids, the transverse and the obliques, have very important biological functions that help us to understand how the muscles are used to regulate loudness. The larynx has the biological responsibility of keeping foreign matter out of the lungs. It does this by closing the vocal folds tightly when a bolus of food enters into the pharynx. This tight closure of the folds is accomplished by contracting the transverse and oblique muscles. This same action is involved in coughing and clearing the throat. When the folds are tightly closed, they allow subglottal pressure to build to very high levels.

We have previously discussed the lateral cricoarytenoids as gentle adductors of the vocal folds. The interarytenoid muscles can also adduct the vocal folds, but they tend to have considerable strength in this action and bring the folds into complete closure. By involving the interarytenoids to some degree in the normal approximation of the folds by the lateral cricoarytenoids, we add some compression to the normal "approximated" position of the vocal folds. This leads to a greater build-up of subglottal air pressure, since it now takes more pressure to overcome the "slightly compressed" folds and set them into vibration. The air stream now leaves the system under greater pressure, and the ear hears increased pressure as an increase in loudness.

The issue of decreased intensity is still another matter. If you will recall from your anatomy classes, the arytenoid cartilages sit on top of the posterior arches of the cricoid cartilage. Contraction of the interarytenoids pulls the arytenoids together, compressing the folds. They also pull the arytenoid cartilages "up hill," up the crest of the cricoid.

When the interarytenoid muscles are relaxed the arytenoid cartilages, because of the natural elasticity of tissue, slide "down hill," or away from each other. Therefore, no muscular action is needed to decrease vocal loudness. This means that we should have less control over decreasing loudness than over increasing loudness. You can test this as follows: Select a pitch and start vocalizing at a low loudness level. Slowly increase the loudness and then slowly decrease the loudness to where you started. Most people will have good control increasing loudness and considerably less control when decreasing it.

THE EXTRINSIC MUSCLES OF THE LARYNX

The are other muscles in the laryngeal region that we should consider. Those found above the hyoid bone are termed the suprahyoids, whereas those below the hyoid bone and just external and anterior to the larynx are called the infrahyoids. We would like to comment about the infrahyoids since, in our opinion, this group of muscles may have a great deal of influence on the performance of the intrinsic muscles of the larynx. These muscles are often referred to as "strap" or "sling" muscles because they tend to strap or sling the larynx in place. These muscles provide protection to the laryngeal system as well as add to its general mobility. During a swallow, for example, they and the suprahyoids are involved in raising the entire larynx and tucking it safely under the protection of the epiglottis. However, during voicing we do not want the strap muscles to contract and pull the larynx up, but only to maintain the degree of contraction necessary to support the larynx. Without going into detail we can simply say that the strength of the extrinsic strap muscles is such that they override and inhibit the fine motor movements of the intrinsic muscles of the larynx. For example, if the strap muscles are contracted, holding the thyroid cartilage firmly in an upward position, the cricothyroid would have little success in adjusting the thyroid cartilage to raise the pitch of the voice. When these muscles are contracted, they reduce the mobility of the larynx and negatively influence voicing, pitch, and loudness.

RESONATION AND AIR FLOW

We are going to approach the vocal mechanics of resonance in a simplified manner. We do not want to delve into the acoustics of resonance, as this is really beyond the scope of this book. Further, in considering the types of clients seen within the clinical environment of the schools, we do not feel it necessary to consider all the subtle types of vocal changes that might be attributable to variations in the size, shape, and coupling of various resonators. Therefore, we will limit our discussion here to the influence of nasal resonance.

The only time that nasal resonance is a necessary part of speech is in the production of the nasal sounds, [m], [n] and [ŋ]. If nasal resonance is not introduced during the production of these sounds, they change to [b], [d] and [g]. For this reason, lack of nasal resonance is viewed by many speech clinicians as an articulation disorder. The voice disorder we are considering here is that of nasal resonance being present in the voice when it is not called for. This could be the extension of nasal resonance beyond the limits of the nasal sound, for example, nasal resonance present throughout the production of the word *hammer*. It might also be the presence of nasal resonance in all speech. In any event, the source of the difficulty is the accessing of the nasal resonator at inappropriate times in speech.

The nasal cavity is the source of nasal resonance. It is isolated from the other resonators in the vocal system by the hard and soft palates. Obviously, if the palate is cleft, the integrity of the system is altered. The nasal cavity cannot be isolated and nasal resonance is present in all speech. In more subtle instances the problem is associated with the movement or the coordination of the movement of the soft palate as it seals off the nasal cavity. In performing this task, the soft palate moves upward and backward to make a seal with the posterior wall of the nasopharynx. At the same time, the back wall of the pharynx is brought slightly forward to meet with the approaching soft palate. These movements must be fast, timed to the occurrence and duration of the nasalized sound, and accurately placed in order to complete the seal. If the seal is accomplished too early or released too soon, the associated sounds are distorted. Also, if the seal is not complete, there will be slight nasal resonance when it should not be occurring.

VOCAL BEHAVIORS

The production of voice is the result of a series of interrelated behaviors performed by an individual. The behaviors are performed in a specific order, each behavior making a necessary contribution before the next behavior occurs. The first behavior is respiration, which provides the power supply for vocal production and contributes to maintaining the power supply over time (checking action) as voicing occurs. The second behavior is phonation. This is a complex behavior that can be divided into two phases, voicing and prosody. Voicing consists of closing the vocal folds in such a way that they can vibrate at their normal frequency. This behavior provides the voice with its basic quality. Prosody consists of muscular adjustments within the larynx that provide the voice with pitch and loudness interaction. The final behavior is that of isolating the nasal resonator for the vocal tract except for those times the system is involved in the production of nasal sounds.

An abnormal system would be any system in which any of the following behavioral problems occur.

1. Inappropriate breathing patterns
2. Inappropriate checking action
3. Inappropriate vocal fold approximation
4. Inappropriate vocal fold vibration
5. Inappropriate laryngeal length, tension, and mass adjustments
6. Inappropriate laryngeal compression adjustments
7. Inappropriate laryngeal adjustment coordination
8. Inappropriate resonance coupling

Any one or any combination of these behavioral deficits can result in a voice disorder by disturbing the vocal quality, pitch, or loudness or any combination thereof.

Chapter 4

Group Therapy

THE SHAPING GROUP

Almost every speech clinician working in a school environment does what is commonly referred to as "group therapy." There are probably as many forms of "group therapy" as there are clinicians. This lack of standardization exists because there are no references the clinician can turn to that set forth guidelines on how to do group therapy. So, each clinician creates her own form of working with a group of clients. Much of the group therapy practiced is really "therapy in a group," individual therapy provided in a group setting. In the school environment, this is partially due to the environmental role models of "teachers" and "students." The clients then play a passive role in therapy, just as they would in the classroom.

The term "group therapy" implies that there is therapeutic interaction between the members of the group, that the group members are involved in both providing therapy for other members of the group and receiving therapy from other group members. During the past 10 years a highly specialized form of group therapy, the shaping group, has been developed for the speech clinician, particularly for the clinician working in the school environment. The operational aspects of the shaping group will be presented in this chapter. There is neither the time nor the space to give a detailed presentation of all aspects of the shaping group in this book. The reader is referred to the chapter, "The Shaping Group: Habituating New Behaviors in the Stutterer" (Leith, 1979) for a detailed presentation of this new form of group therapy. More general discussions of the shaping group are to be found in other books and articles by Leith (1982, 1984). In these other references you will find that four different shaping groups are defined. In this book we have reduced the types of shaping groups to three because of limited age range of voice clients the school clinician deals with.

CONTRASTS BETWEEN
GROUP THERAPY FORMS

In the more traditional therapy in a group, as the clinician works with a member of the group, the other group members listen and watch the therapy as they are waiting their turn. All modeling, guidance and information are provided by the speech clinician. She also evaluates all of the responses of the clients and administers the rewards and penalties. Interaction between group members is at a minimum. Learning occurs with each group member only when they are receiving therapy from the clinician.

By contrast, all members of the shaping group are actively involved in therapy at all times. The group members, whenever possible, join in providing the modeling, guidance, and information for each other. Judgments of the responses and the application of either reward or penalty are also shared by the group members. All group members are expected to be both clinicians and clients. They act as clinicians when the group is focusing on another group member, and are clients when the group focuses on them. Since they are always involved in the therapeutic interaction, they are always involved in a learning experience.

LEARNING FUNCTIONS OF THE SHAPING GROUP

One of the most important things that a client must learn in therapy is to monitor his own speech. If he does not have this skill, there will be no carry-over of the new speech or vocal behavior to outside environments. The client must be aware of when and if the old behavior is occurring so that he can make the necessary corrections in order for the new behavior to occur. In more traditional group therapy in which the clinician makes all decisions regarding the correctness of the member's behaviors and administers the rewards and penalties, the members of the group have little opportunity to learn to monitor speech or voice. The issue of listening skills is addressed only when the individual group member is receiving his therapy. One of the focal points of the shaping group is the training of all group members' listening skills.

Shaping group members are expected to monitor not only their own speech but also to monitor the speech of the other group members. They learn to monitor their own speech not only to achieve the rewards from the group but also to avoid group penalty. They monitor the speech of other members in order to apply either a reward or a penalty. Self-monitoring skills are carefully taught in the shaping group. This makes the generalization of the new speech behavior to other environments much easier and faster.

The shaping group also provides its members with an opportunity to use their new speech behavior in a semisocial environment where the basic speech form is conversational. The client can practice his new speech behavior with a group of people, talking on a variety of subjects. The group members will provide him with honest feedback in terms of how effective he is in using the new speech behavior.

The shaping group provides the opportunity to create "role playing" dealing with situations in which a group member may be having a particularly difficult time. If a group member must give an oral report in class, the group can serve as the "class" while the client gives his oral report, using his new speech behavior. Other members of the group could use the group to "practice" talking in a variety of speaking situations that might be stressful to one of the group members. This aspect of the group function represents the gradual introduction of an S— where the S— is so strong that the client is unable to use his new vocal behavior.

WHEN TO USE THE SHAPING GROUP

When we consider the three basic steps in therapy, getting the new behavior to occur, stabilizing the new behavior, and generalizing the new behavior, the shaping group is most effective in the last two steps. This does not mean that it can not be used in the first step, only that there will be a mixture of therapy in a group and shaping group during this step. If all of the clients who are to make up the shaping group are new clients, the clinician will have to do some individual therapy with each client until their new behavior is beginning to occur. The process can then shift to the shaping group. If only one new client is introduced to an ongoing shaping group, a variation in group organization to be discussed later in the chapter will allow this client to receive individual attention without disrupting the ongoing group. Each speech clinician will determine when the shaping group works best for her, considering the number of clients she is working with, her time schedule, and other factors.

THE CLINICIAN'S ROLE
AS SHAPING GROUP LEADER

The role of shaping group leader is quite different from the activities the clinician performs in therapy in a group. She is no longer a "clinician" in the strictest sense of the word in that she is not involved in the direct provision of therapy. She is now involved in training the members of the group to function as clinicians for themselves and the other group members. This training is accomplished through modeling, guidance, and information provided by the speech clinician. She is still adhering to the CIM model because she is still teaching. However, she is now teaching behaviors other than speech behaviors. As the group members learn to function as "clinicians" in the shaping group, the clinician withdraws her stimuli (modeling, guidance, and information) and assumes a different role. With the group members maintaining the therapeutic interaction of the group, the clinician can now become more of an observer, a moderator, an orchestrator. She continues to carefully monitor the group interaction and therapy, only intervening when necessary. Her role is more passive than active, and the majority of talking is done by the group members rather than by the clinician. For many clinicians, this has proven to be the most difficult aspect of assuming the role of shaping group leader, to be quiet and not monopolize the group interaction. It is foreign to us to allow the clients to perform their own therapy, even under our strict guidance. But it does work, more effectively in many cases since the clients are usually more demanding of themselves than the clinician.

TYPES OF SHAPING GROUPS

In order to accommodate age differences in groups, three levels of shaping groups have been established. Each group level is unique in that the clients at each level have different needs, social maturity, and cognitive maturity. The three levels of groups are the elementary shaping group, the junior shaping group, and the senior/adult shaping group.

Elementary Shaping Group

Typically, children between the ages of 5 and 11 years make up this group. Further, a 3 year age range among the group members should be maintained. The size of the group should be limited, if possible, to three children, since children of this age lack the social maturity to interact with larger groups. The male/female ratio in the younger groups is not important but does begin to affect the group interaction at the upper end of the age range. These are only guidelines, not hard and fast rules. The maturity of each client is also a factor the clinician must consider when assigning clients to groups.

Junior Shaping Group

The junior shaping group is formed with children between the ages of 12 and 15 years. Owing to increased social maturity, the group can function with four members with a 4 year range of ages between group members. The clinician must keep in mind that she is now dealing with clients who are entering the strange age of puberty. This is going to have a direct effect on the age range of the group, the group size, and the male/female ratio, which now becomes an important factor. Decisions about the make-up of the group must be made by the clinician involved with the group. In making the decisions she must consider the client's ages, their degree of social maturity, and how they relate to the opposite sex. There must be careful planning with this group, and the clinician will find her role as group leader a bit more complicated. This is a sensitive age for the clients, and group interactions may tend to be a bit more difficult to initiate and control.

Senior/Adult Shaping Group

The ages of clients involved in this group is somewhat dependent on the local rules governing who is eligible for clinical services. We will base our group on the upper limit of 24 years of age. Therefore, this group may consist of clients between the ages of 16 and 24 years. With this wide an age span, we would want to limit the range of ages within a group to no more than 4 years. We will also attempt to limit the size of the group to four members. The male/female ratio is not as important with this shaping group but the clinician must make some decisions in this regard according to the maturity of the clients. If the clinician has a mature group of clients, the group size can be increased to five.

ACTIVITIES OF GROUP MEMBERS

The Clients

The shaping group cannot operate efficiently without total group interaction. This involves monitoring of the speech behaviors of other group members, administering rewards or penalties, and participating in group discussions. Regardless of whether the group is homogeneous or heterogeneous, the members of the group must know what behaviors all other members are working on. If they are to reward or penalize behavioral performances, they must know how well the behaviors can be performed. This information is provided during the formation of the group as the clinician identifies each group member and what behavior they are working on. If some group members are more advanced in therapy, they can demonstrate their new behaviors. Members who are just starting therapy will probably have to receive individual attention in the group until the new behavior is beginning to occur. This will help identify the new behavior for the other members of the group. The group members can then become involved in shaping the behavior to the behavior change goal.

This process of identification of behavior change goals forms the base of improving listen skills, since the group members must then listen to and identify a variety of speech behaviors. The clients are being taught to listen to both *what* is said and *how* it is said. All of this is fundamental to self-monitoring and this is the basic skill needed for carry-over of the new speech behaviors to other speaking environments. As the monitoring skills improve, so will the speech performance of the group members.

The group leader will have to specifically train the group members to administer rewards and penalties. This is a new behavior for them. They can be taught this new behavior through information provided by the group leader as well as through the modeling provided by both the group leader and the other members of the group. The most important source of modeling will be the group leader, and she should explain both what she is doing and why she is doing it. It is extremely important that the group leader explain that group members can help one another through rewards and penalties. The reward concept will not be difficult to explain but the penalty concept will offer some challenges. We have found it helpful to explain this in terms of "feedback." A group member can not change a behavior if he is not aware of when he is performing it incorrectly. The member needs both types of "feedback," rewards when he does it correctly and penalties when he does it incorrectly. Again, the penalty we are talking about is not severe. It is more in the form of letting the person know that what they did was not correct or acceptable.

In that all members of the shaping group are involved in administering both rewards and penalties, these contingent events are quite strong. The shaping group members make up a "peer" group and this takes on added significance when rewards or penalties are administered. Because the group members are operating in "peer" social interaction, they have strong approach motivation to receive rewards from their peers. A strong avoidance motivation to avoid being penalized by their peer group is also present.

The Clinician

The role of group leader calls for some new behaviors on the part of the clinician. She is no longer a clinician working in an individual therapy setting. She is now guiding a therapeutic interaction, acting as a moderator when the needs arises. She is more of a supervisor than an active clinician. Let us examine some of the tasks the group leader must assume. The clinician models:

1. The administration of rewards
2. The administration of penalty
3. The performance of new speech behaviors for new group members
4. The various tasks that make up the role of the group leader
5. The participation and interaction in group activities

The clinician provides guidance for:

1. The group members in determining rewards and penalties to be administered in the group
2. The group interaction to prevent it from drifting away from therapy
3. The group interaction to maintain a balance of rewards and penalties so the group does not become either too positive or too negative
4. The group interaction so that no members receive too many penalties
5. The group requirements for behavioral performance for rewards so that they are within the member's capabilities

—NOTES—

The clinician provides information about:

1. The individual group members' behavior change goals
2. The operational rules for the shaping group
3. The purpose of applying rewards or penalties to other members of the group

OPERATING THE SHAPING GROUP

Instructions

The first step in creating a shaping group is to set forth the rules and regulations of the group. All members of the group must understand how the group will operate and what they are expected to do as a member of the group. The clinician should stress that all members must participate in the group interactions. Included in this information are the reasons for using rewards and penalties. It would be advisable to discuss this with the group members after the information has been presented to make sure that everyone understood what he had been told.

Identification of Behavior Change Goals

With any kind of heterogeneous or homogeneous group, the clinician should identify and describe the behavior change goal of each group member and, if possible, have the group member demonstrate their proficiency with the new behavior. All behavior change goals should be clearly understood by the group members before proceeding. A group discussion of behavior change goals would be in order here. This is an essential part of starting the shaping group, because the effectiveness of the group is dependent on the application of rewards and penalties to the appropriate behaviors.

Rewards and Penalties

Before the group interaction can begin, a decision must be made as to what will be used as a reward and as a penalty. The same reward and penalty must be used for all group members. The group leader and the group members must decide on what would be rewarding and what would be penalizing. Verification of the reward and penalty will be made by the group leader in observing the effects of the rewards and penalties on the behaviors once the group commences. The group leader should not decide on the reward and the penalty without input from the group members. Some guidelines for selecting the reward and penalty would include such factors as ease of application, not too time consuming, and not disruptive of the group interaction. A token economy will satisfy all of these requirements. There is also no problem with the actual reward, since there can be a variety of back-up rewards for the group members to select from.

If other forms of rewards and penalties are used, consider that with visual events, the recipient must be looking at the individual to be aware of it. This is quite difficult in a group situation. However, one group waved small white flags for reward and red flags for penalty and it worked very well. Auditory signals seem better adapted to this kind of clinical interaction. However, the auditory signals probably should not be verbal phrases such as "That was good" or "That was not very good." If presented during a group interaction, they interrupt the therapy. A group might consider such things as a hand clap for reward and a finger snap for penalty. Other rewards and penalties to consider are a cough, clearing the throat, a tongue click, the words *yes* and *no*, and various noisemakers. The danger here is that the noise level of reward or penalty can interfere with the group activities.

Getting the Group Started

The group interaction can begin after the instructions are given, the group members' behaviors identified, and the reward and penalty determined. We will discuss a particular group since there are so many possible combinations of shaping groups. We will discuss an elementary shaping group made up of clients with a variety of disorders. Each client can produce his or her new speech behavior on a more or less regular basis. The voice client in the group is working on stabilizing a new pitch level. All members of the group are still dependent on the reward for the speech performance. The group is reward oriented as it begins. The group starts by having the members discuss a neutral but interesting topic, such as vacations or hobbies. Each member is asked to make a comment on the topic. As each member speaks, the clinician provides some form of guidance to prompt the new behaviors. With the voice client she might give a gesture that indicates, "Lower your pitch." When the client speaks, using his new pitch, she rewards him for his new speech behavior, modeling the giving of a reward for the other group members. She continues to model rewarding new speech behaviors, encouraging other group members to join her. When a group member rewards another member for a new speech behavior, she in turn rewards him for his new rewarding behavior. She is rewarding the member for his monitoring and rewarding of another group member's speech. She wants to encourage members to reward one another, so the rewarding behavior is itself rewarded when it occurs. The group process is operational when the group members begin to reward each other for their new speech behaviors. At this time the clinician fades her modeling, allowing the group members to provide their own modeling. The clinician then assumes the role of group leader, monitoring and guiding.

Penalty should not be introduced into the group until the group process is stable, with all members participating in the discussions and rewarding each other. Penalty is particularly useful as the group members become more engrossed in the discussion topics. They become more interested in *what* they are saying as opposed to *how* they are saying it. They then tend to "forget" their new speech behavior. For example, the voice client becomes so involved in telling about his vacation that he forgets to maintain his new pitch level. Another member catches this and penalizes him, perhaps by removing a token. This reminds the client to use his new pitch. At the same time, the clinician rewards the group member for catching the voice client's use of his old pitch. This is another monitoring behavior the clinician wants to encourage so it is rewarded. It is extremely important to remember that an incorrect behavior is only penalized when we are certain that the client can produce the correct behavior.

VARIATIONS IN GROUP ORGANIZATION

When the group is stable and operating effectively, group members should be trained to act as group leader. The clinician has provided the model of the group leader and she now allows a group member to lead the group while she provides guidance. This group member is then providing a model of the group leader for the other members of the group. The clinician can then fade her group leader role and assume other roles. When group members can assume the group leader role, the clinician is free to organize the group in several different ways.

With a group in which a member needs individual attention or in which a new member is just starting therapy, the group can continue to operate with a member group leader while the clinician provides the individual therapy. The group should not continue under the direction of a member group leader over an extended period of time.

From time to time the clinician should withdraw from all group interaction and observe the shaping group in operation. These "objective" observations are important so that both individual members and group interactions can be carefully observed. The clinician is free to do this if she has trained a group member to lead the group while she observes. This gives her the opportunity to evaluate the progress of each group member, make changes in the group organization if warranted, and determine if the group is working toward the proper goals of therapy.

In the event that it is impossible to limit the group size to that recommended here, there is still another variation of the shaping group that will solve this problem. An elementary shaping group of six members has too many members for the group to operate effectively. In this instance the clinician selects three group members to form a shaping group. The other members are then assigned to serve as individual monitors to the three members of the shaping group. The monitors sit behind their "clients" and monitor their speech. Their job is to remind their "client" to use his new speech behavior when he enters the group discussion. They also provide rewards and penalties to their "clients." Although not directly involved in the group interaction, the monitors practice their listening skills as they monitor their "client's" speech. When the roles are reversed among the members of the shaping group, the additional practice in listening skills will be manifested in more consistent use of the client's new behaviors. By using group members as monitors, all members of the group are still involved in therapy and not "waiting" for their turn.

ADDING NEW MEMBERS TO A GROUP

A shaping group started at the beginning of the school year is an ongoing procedure. As members achieve their behavior change goal and are dismissed from therapy, new members are added. New members must be introduced to the operational guidelines of the group, the behavior change goals of the various group members, and the reward and penalty system and the reasons for using it. The remaining group members should provide this information under the guidance of the clinician. This is a good review for the remaining members. All this information can be presented in one meeting of the group. As the group resumes therapy, the new member learns to function as a group member through the modeling and guidance provided by the other group members. In this way, new members can constantly be added to an ongoing group.

THE CIM AND THE SHAPING GROUP

You should recognize that the CIM is the basis of the shaping group interactions. However, the stimulus now comes from a member of the group, perhaps in the form of a question. The member to whom the question was directed will think about it and then respond. This member's response is the stimulus for the group to evaluate and respond to. The reward or the penalty is very strong both because it comes from a "peer" group and because of the number of peers involved in administering it. The strength of the rewarda or penalties may vary from application to application. If there are three members of the group evaluating a response, they may not all agree that it should be rewarded or penalized. If only one member provides the reward, the reward is not very strong. Rewards from two group members are stronger, and a reward from all three members is the strongest. This concept of strength of group reaction also applies to the application of a penalty.

An important task of the group leader during group interactions is to monitor the attending behaviors of the group members. If a group member's attention is waning, the clinician can focus the group on his attending behaviors for rewards or penalties.

Another very important clinical feature of the shaping group is that all group members assume specific stimulus roles. As they present rewards they become an S+ for the other group members. The S− role stems from applying penalty. These special stimulus roles are carried over outside the clinical environment. This means that when group members encounter each other in the school, they will "cue up" the correct behaviors and discourage the incorrect behaviors. This important function of the shaping group is a great asset in generalizing the new behaviors to other environments in the school.

Chapter 5

Interpersonal Communication and Counseling

INTRODUCTION

Our profession is in a period of attempting to increase objectivity and accountability in the treatment of communication disorders. Our competence/performance approach to evaluation and treatment and our emphasis on vocal behaviors is a reflection of that recent professional emphasis. Although this important period has produced numerous diagnostic tests, innovative clinical procedures, and technical hardware to enhance our clinical effectiveness, it has also in some ways re-emphasized the importance of client/clinician relationships in the therapy process. We sense that clinicians have a renewed respect for the importance of knowing the client and the client's family beyond the objective and accountable descriptors found in the client's file. There appears to be a renewed recognition of interpersonal communication and counseling as factors necessary for meaningful therapy. People enter the helping professions, including speech therapy, with a genuine concern for the quality of life for others. This attribute of caring is essential to the therapy process and is generally thought of as the *humanistic* aspect of clinical work. This chapter attempts to confront the issue of humanism in voice therapy by examining two important aspects of therapy, interpersonal communication and counseling. All of these interactions are based on the Clinical Interaction Model (CIM) presented in Chapter 2.

Counseling, in its broadest sense, is not a new clinical aspect of therapy. Think of the many treatment programs for the stuttering client. These programs have historically involved working with the client's perceptions of himself and others in the modification of his dysfluencies. In voice therapy, there is a long history of treating voice disorders associated with emotional causes with a counseling approach. Yet, the word "counseling" somehow suggests to many clinicians that their work

—NOTES—

is extending beyond their training and into other professional fields. If it is the word "counseling" that is bothersome, then let us agree that what we are talking about under the counseling label is client/clinician communication. Improvement in our client/clinician interpersonal communication can significantly help us in providing therapy. In particular, effective communication and counseling is a natural part of appropriate therapy. It is also critical to the carry-over process and essential to the understanding of the client's various speaking environments.

Advantages to Improved Interpersonal Communication and Counseling

Before we address the application of improved communication with the voice-disordered client, we would like to discuss the positive influence that good interpersonal communication and counseling can have on therapy.

Communication and Counseling Saves Time in Therapy. Good therapy involves appropriate and meaningful tasks that are best structured by understanding the client's likes and dislikes, fears, attitudes, beliefs, and motivations. We are not speaking about the process of establishing rapport, which is very important in all clinical work, but rather we are suggesting that the efficiency of therapy can be significantly increased by spending time communicating with your client.

Communication and Counseling Aids in the Generalization Process. It is often noted that one of our greatest problems in therapy is getting a new behavior to occur outside of the clinical speaking environment. Communication and counseling can be an effective tool in understanding the client's environment and how our therapy fits into that environment. We cannot rectify the lack of generalization of a new behavior if we have not taken the time to understand the client's speaking environment.

Communication and Counseling Indicates to the Client That We Care about Him As Well As His Communication Problem. We, as clinicians, must be certain that the client does not feel that we are only interested in the communication problem and not in the client himself. Clients respond best to clinicians who treat them first as individuals and second as clients. Opening and closing statements for a therapy session should convey this important message. The opening statement, "How have you been?" is more humanistic than "How has your speech been?"

Communication and Counseling Involves the Family and Significant Others. Parents of children with communication disorders have many fears concerning their child's potential. Remember that our clients spend more hours with their families than they do with us, and if a child perceives that his parents are fearful about his speech, these perceptions may serve as roadblocks to our therapy. When the child knows that there is communication between his parents and the clinician, he is likely to have a more positive attitude toward therapy. Furthermore, if we have communicated with the family throughout the therapy program, they are ready for their role when we need their help and cooperation.

Communication and Counseling Establishes Improved Client/Clinician Relationships. The clinical environment must to be conducive to the learning process. Taking the time to establish a positive human relationship will produce the respect and cooperation needed for the changing or modifying of a client's behavior. If a child enjoys his therapy, we have increased the likelihood that he will be cooperative. When a client is cooperative, we increase the efficiency of our therapy. Taking the time to establish a positive human working relationship can sometimes be the difference between successful and unsuccessful therapy.

THE VOICE DISORDERED CLIENT

Each communication disorder has unique characteristics that are important for clinicians to understand if they are to provide appropriate therapy. To start with, the voice disordered client is rarely self-referred. Both children and adults may react with surprise at the suggestion that their voice may be in need of therapy. Statements such as "I have always talked like this" are common reactions. In your early contacts with the client you should not attempt to convince him that he has a voice problem, but rather you should attempt to show him how important voice is in effective communication.

The client may actually resist any attempt you make to modify his vocal production. We have a strong suspicion that many children and adults equate their voice with their personality. This then becomes the basis of rejecting changing their voice, even when the voice is clearly below expected standards. However, we need to remember that some unusual voices, even "bad" voices, are the source of praise and recognition for their owners. The child who has learned how to talk like a frog may get considerable reinforcement from his peers for his voice. If you change the way a client sounds you may be changing their self-concept. This relationship between voice and personality is understandable when we think of the number of ways in which the voice carries significant emotional information; for example, the "shaky" voice is associated with nervousness. Because the voice carries so many of the prosodics of language, it reflects the client's fears, doubts, anger, happiness, and other emotions.

The voice client, then, often comes to us as the result of a referral, not convinced that he has a problem, or he may come to us and have a genuine fear that successful therapy may change his personality, or he may come to us knowing that his voice is a source of irritation to some but pleasure to others. These common factors associated with the voice disordered client, plus the host of other factors each individual brings to the therapy environment, should underscore that effective interpersonal communication and counseling are essential to voice therapy.

There are, of course, voice disorders that are directly related to a psychological cause. These disorders are most often found in adult clients and are best treated with a counseling approach. This chapter will not deal with those disorders of voice because of their rarity in children. They do remind us, however, that the relationship between the voice and the psyche is very powerful for some. Our goal for the remainder of this chapter is to provide information on the ways clinicians can improve their interpersonal communication. We will also present two counseling strategies: direct and indirect counseling techniques.

INTERPERSONAL COMMUNICATION

The concept of "helping" is a basic ingredient in all interpersonal communication. When we stress the fact that therapy is a helping function, the focus of improving our interpersonal skills becomes clear. Some of the most important ingredients necessary to improve the communication between client and clinician are:

1. *Empathy.* Empathy allows the clinician to think *with* the client rather than *for* or *about* the client. The clinician attempts to place herself in the internal frame of reference of the client rather than to remain outside or aloof from the client's perception. However, too much empathy can be dangerous, and too little will place serious constraints on the communication process.

2. *Caring.* When the clinician cares about the client, their relationship is warm and friendly. Human behaviors such as smiling, attending, and appropriate eye contact can indicate to the client that the clinician cares about him. The ability to show warmth and caring is often critical during the early stages of therapy. As with empathy, too much caring can be a problem, whereas too little

sends the message of coolness and detachment.

3. *Respect*. It is important that clinicians make certain that clients know we respect them. Respect indicates to clients that we care about them as individuals beyond their communication needs. Respect is usually fostered when our words and deeds match and when we are predictable and consistent in our relations with our clients.

4. *Openness*. Successful interpersonal communication is often dependent upon respect, and respect or trust is usually built upon open sharing by the two communicators. Others have described this aspect of interpersonal communication as "genuineness." The ability to be open or genuine in our communication with our clients builds trust, and trust is essential in the teaching and learning process.

5. *Competence*. The client must feel confident that the person they entrust their communication disorder to is competent. There are many ways that clinicians can build interpersonal competence. Experience is the best teacher in achieving interpersonal competence. One way to quickly improve interpersonal communication is to attempt to be concrete and specific with your communication. Although it may be appropriate at times to allow the client to wander verbally, the clinician should try to keep her verbalization focused on the clinical interaction and the goal.

In addition to these brief observations about the skills that are important to improving interpersonal communication, we would like to examine three other factors: the power of words, honesty in interpersonal communication and therapy, and listening skills.

The Power of Words

Words are very powerful tools. Although it is impossible to obtain complete agreement on the meanings of words, interpersonal communication strives to relate feelings, emotions, and experiences with as much accuracy as possible. The sage advice that emerges from the study of words (general semantics) is "Say what you mean, and mean what you say," to which most counselors reply, "That's easy for you to say." We would advise the speech clinician to think very carefully about the words she is using and the way she is presenting them. When the client is talking, the clinician should focus on what he said and what he *really* meant to say. The clinician can always ask the communication partner, "Did you understand what I just said?" or "Can you tell me in your words what I just said?" In addition, clinicians can ask their com-

—NOTES—

munication partner, "Did I understand you to say that . . .?" or "Let me put into my words what I think you said." If this effort to clarify meaning appears unnecessary, we ask you to tape record a few of your therapy sessions and make a count of the number of times that the communication process may have broken down because of a lack of agreement on the meanings of the words used.

Clinicians are often advised to restrict their use of professional vocabulary when working with clients or families. The behavioral orientation will help in that it deals with very specific behaviors and tends not to depend on vague auditory descriptors or confusing medical terms. It is important to note that this does not mean that you "talk down" to a client, that is, speak to a client, regardless of age, as though the client were a child. Again, a tape recording of your therapy will give you insight. Listen to yourself and, when appropriate, note where changes can be made to improve your communication style.

Honesty

A common complaint from clients and families about our profession and other education and health professions is the lack of candor from the professional. Such common phrases as "He'll grow out of it" or "Let's just wait and see for a few months" are often nothing more than a cover for our lack of ability to communicate effectively with clients and families. Clients and families have the right to know *everything* that we know about the problem and the appropriateness of our remedial choices. For example, when we the authors conduct a voice evaluation, we show the client each entry that we have made. We ask them if they understand each task and what it measured. We explain all of our assessments, interpret all of our findings, and reveal much of our thinking. We find that clients of all ages feel good about being included in the evaluation process. They also often gain a good grasp of the steps we will follow in therapy. In therapy, the same commitment to inform the client and family should be used. When the client understands the task he is to perform, why it is important to perform that task, and how this will improve the voice, the client demonstrates additional commitment to the therapy process.

Learning to Listen

One unfortunate by-product of organized, efficient, and accountable therapy is that we often forget to include listening as part of the therapy. Evaluations, therapy, and working with families are essentially communication processes. The best form of communication in these activities is two-way communication or dialogue between clinician and client. Basic to any communication or dialogue is listening. Good listening requires the clinician to listen for the total meaning of the message, which includes both the surface content and the undersurface intent of the speaker. Following are some factors for the clinician to consider when attempting to improve her listening skill:

1. *Fear.* When the clinician fears for her safety, health, or even her position of authority, the ability to listen is reduced. If a parent was to suddenly approach a clinician in anger regarding his or her child, the clinician's ability to accurately decode the parent's message is limited. Allowing the parent to fully express anger without the clinician's entering into the debate (usually about her professional competence or judgment) solves two problems: It allows for a normal emotion,anger,to be vented and it allows for the communication process to return to better encoding and decoding. In most clinical situations the angry parent is not genuinely angry with the clinician. Rather, the parent is in the stage of anger associated with grieving or the anger is over the lack of communication from the professional community. If a parent is angry with the clinician, it is very possible that he or she actually likes her and trusts his or her anger to her. After the clinician allows parents or clients to express anger, they can begin to put additional value on the message that is being delivered. Knowing this may allow clinicians to place less importance on information obtained during fearful conditions.

2. *Intimacy.* The clinician can often care about and be emotionally involved with the client and his family beyond the typical professional level. The fear of rejection or eventual detachment may cause the clinician to distort incoming messages. In this example, we "hear" what we want to hear rather than the message. To some extent the opposite is also true. Caring about the communicator allows us to listen with additional enthusiasm and attention. We need to care about our clients while avoiding feelings of intimacy.

3. *Feelings.* Often clinicians respond to a strong message before giving themselves an opportunity to reflect on the message itself. Most counseling requires that the professional enter the therapy session value-free. If we bring strong opinions and values to the act of listening, then we can often respond reflexively and judgmentally rather than thoughtfully. When the clinician "hears" a message that is offensive, the best advice is to count slowly and silently to ten before responding. Silence allows the sender to modify the statement, and it allows the clinician to respond with vocabulary that

is not judgmental, critical, or self-serving. The act of being a good listener does not guarantee that what you hear will all be pleasant, but it does require that you listen carefully (often nonjudgmentally) before responding.

4. *Distractions*. Good listening can be very difficult in some environments. When the surroundings are full of distractions, good listening becomes difficult or impossible. Room arrangement, adequate time allotment and consideration of the client's needs can be very helpful. Remember, when the environment is not conducive to good listening, the message may be poorly decoded.

The good listener's nonverbal body language matches the listening intent and the verbal response. Clinicians are reminded that the youngest and most naive of their clients know if the clinician is paying attention or cares about what he says. Parents also know if the clinician wants to communicate. Sometimes our desire to be efficient and accountable appears to be at odds with the humanistic calling of helping professions. We encourage you to invest the time to listen to your client and his family. It will result in more efficient and effective therapy.

COUNSELING

This section of the chapter does not propose to identify or resolve any of the counseling needs the voice client may have. Our purpose is to remind you of the integrity of the individual client and his family. Counseling is not a special dimension of therapy always managed by other professionals but rather is a natural aspect of therapy that many clients with voice disorders need. Remember that therapy involves human communication and interaction and that we work with *people* who have disorders, not just with disorders.

Indirect Counseling

At times the client's problem demands that we incorporate counseling as a partner to voice therapy or, in other instances, as the major focus of therapy. Recognizing the client's or family's need for counseling is not as difficult as it may initially seem. First, we have found that parents of children with any handicap may experience the various stages associated with mourning. Some people feel that mourning is only associated with a major and critical loss. However, we have found parents in deep mourning because their child had an articulation disorder while parents of children with serious multiple handicaps in the same counseling group had less of a sense of loss.

Clinicians often wonder just what parents are mourning about. All parents hope for the "perfect" child. But when the parents are told that their child has a communication disorder, an imperfection, the parents may view this as evidence that their hope for perfection has been lost. Loss is almost always the factor that produces mourning. Mourning and the stages associated with the grieving process are well documented. What should be remembered is that mourning is a natural mental process (healing) for dealing with loss. Often the person going through mourning may say or do things that seem unusual to the nongriever. Denial, guilt, depression, anger, bargaining, and accepting reality are labels given to the many stages and feeling parents can go through as they come to grips with the loss of the perfect child that they had hoped for. These stages can also occur for spouses or any family member who had a plan for the future changed by a diagnosis. Given that parental cooperation is a critical agent in most therapy with children, clinicians need to appreciate that the parents themselves may need support before they can contribute significantly to the therapy process. How does the clinician help? First, clinicians must recognize that mourning is a normal and natural process. Second, clinicians can provide the one form of help that seems to speed the healing process, *listening*. Finally, the clinician can provide the opportunity to remove the barriers to the communication process. She can have monthly sessions with the parents of her clients, provide for fathers- or mothers-only meetings, or even have sessions with siblings and any significant others. In this instance, the clinician would not be providing therapy but rather would be providing the opportunity for the parents and family to express their feelings and emotions during the healing process.

Indirect therapy is the process of allowing the clients and others involved with the client the opportunity to express their feelings and emotions, knowing that the expression of those feelings will help them "work out" the problem. Indirect therapy does not assume that the client has a problem that needs direct intervention but that the client has a problem that only he can work through, providing someone cares enough to listen. The client (or others) may make unusual statements such as "I hate my mother" or "Sometimes I hate my son." The clinician should listen, clarify the statement, or say to the client, "Tell me more about those feelings." We have observed clinicians use fewer than 50 words during an hour session, and then heard the clients, upon leaving, thank the clinician for helping them.

—NOTES—

The keys to successful indirect counseling are

1. Reveal that you genuinely care.
2. Be a good listener.
3. Be a value-free listener.
4. Accept the mourning process as normal.
5. Provide the opportunity for communication.

Direct Counseling

Direct counseling is actually guidance communication. Sometimes we encounter clients and families that are not grieving but lack the guidance necessary to complete essential tasks. For one reason or another, the client cannot seem to complete important tasks, such as home assignments in therapy. These clients always have excuses for their inability to finish an assignment. The pattern of lack of follow-through is often found in other aspects of their schoolwork or life. These clients need a directed approach that follows the precepts of Reality Therapy (Glasser, 1965).

The basic goal of directed counseling is to help the client learn how to be successful. These clients frequently present a history of a lack of knowing how to reach desired goals through a step-by-step process. After initial sessions of indirect intervention, the clinician establishes a firm, businesslike approach to guidance and therapy. The clinician and client establish one attainable goal that is to be accomplished before the next session. When the client comes to the next session, the first task is to review the assignment. Any failure to complete the task is rejected. A compromise or new goal is established and the client is expected to complete the new task. These assignments are usually written in the form of a *contract* and signed by both the clinician and the client. Continued failure to meet the contract may result, where applicable, in the cancellation of therapy. Success with the contract results in a reward and a joint discussion of a new, equally demanding contract. What is essentially being taught and learned is responsibility. The tasks should be related to the therapy process.

It has been our experience that many clients do not understand responsibility. Without client responsibility, most therapy programs are not going to succeed. The clinician presents a caring but firm link in the learning process. Consistency of expectation is paramount. Once the client is demonstrating the ability to achieve agreed-upon contracts, the clinician may move the contracts into areas beyond voice therapy. The reason that the client needs to expand into other behavior areas is to complete the learning of how to succeed. The choice of goals for the contract should be mutually agreed upon. Generous praise is given for successful contracts, but the praise is for commitment rather than for the task itself.

Directed therapy is the process of teaching the client values and expectations that are common to the society of which he is a part. Direct counseling assumes a basic community standard and ethic of behavior. These are often difficult for some clients to approach because they have a history of failure. They have alibis for their failures and the alibis have been accepted. Direct counseling is often needed for older children and young adults who have a history of failure in school and have adopted the failure syndrome.

The keys to successful direct counseling are

1. Reveal that you genuinely care.
2. Be unwilling to accept excuses for inappropriate behavior.
3. Be willing to express both your values and the prevailing community values.
4. Reject the concept that failure is explainable.
5. Provide the opportunity to develop success by developing contracts that the client can succeed with.

We are including a therapy approach in this chapter because we want you, the reader, to realize that interpersonal communication and counseling can be applied in a unique form of therapy, client-directed therapy. The basic tenant of this therapy approach assumes that the client and the clinician have established good communication and respect for each other. After indirect or direct counseling has produced a positive working relationship, the clinician asks the client to join her in selecting the appropriate therapy intervention. The clinician takes the necessary time to explain all the factors that make up a normal voice, how a normal voice might become abnormal, and how therapy is usually done. The clinician, for example, asks the client to rate his vocal parameters for their adequacy. The parameters might include vocal fold approximation and synchrony, vocal pitch, loudness, prosody, and resonance. The client then selects the parameter that he believes needs to be modified. Even if the client selects a parameter that the clinician does not feel is the primary therapy need, therapy is planned around the parameter selected by the client. If the client is incorrect, joint evaluations should reveal the mistake and discussions should continue for the selection of a new parameter. What might be considered a "waste of time" in fact may save valuable therapy time. The approach promotes participation by the client in changing his voice. The approach reveals a respect by the clinician for the values and opinions of the client. Finally, when the client improves his understanding of how the

—NOTES—

voice works and what the significant parameters of the voice are, he often provides insight into the problem that may be of significant value.

The competence/performance voice evaluation is a logical tool to use with client directed therapy since it identifies the important behaviors of voice and measures those behaviors in isolation and in combined vocal performances.

The keys to successful client directed therapy are

1. Use indirect communication and counseling to establish genuineness.
2. Include the client as a full partner in therapy.
3. Teach the client the parameters of normal voice.
4. Allow the client to select the direction of therapy.
5. Allow the client to determine success of therapy.

Section II
The Pretherapy
Process

Chapter 6

The Voice Evaluation

EVALUATING VOCAL PERFORMANCE

What is a voice evaluation? A voice evaluation is the process of collecting information about a client and his voice. The data can be collected directly from the client, indirectly from someone associated with the client, objectively with an instrument, or subjectively in the form of our sensory classifications or cognitive opinions. Once the information is collected, it is arranged in a logical order or sequence, analyzed, and compared with the information we have on normal voice production. We then reach certain conclusions and make a statement of our findings. This statement may be an appraisal of the voice, ranging from normal voice production to a severe vocal disorder. The statement may also be in the form of a diagnosis, indicating what you believe the cause of the disorder to be. Finally, the statement may take the form of a differential diagnosis, suggesting a probable cause by eliminating other possible causes. With this statement you may also suggest diagnostic therapy in order to gather additional information to support your causal, or etiological, statement.

There are two main reasons why we spend so much valuable clinical time performing an evaluation. First, the evaluation assists us in our ability to communicate effectively with ourselves and with other professionals about the disorder. It provides us with a frame of reference and a vocabulary. When we establish a cause, it gives us a way to approach the body of knowledge associated with that particular cause. Second, the evaluation provides us with a basis on which to plan our therapy. If our therapy is directed at specific vocal behaviors, we must have a adequate assessment of the performance of the behaviors in order to determine both our behavior change goal and the means of accomplishing the goal.

Our profession in general depends heavily on subjective instead of objective data. We rely to a great extent on judgments based on what we hear rather than on judgments based on what we measure, either with electronic instruments or in the form of a standardized test. Most evaluations utilize both subjective and objective data, including the voice evaluation procedure that follows. As clinicians, we must recognize that there are no instruments available to us that replace the professional judgment we make as we auditorily and cognitively monitor our clients. Indeed, some instruments will supplement our cognitive judgment but they still do not replace our professional opinion.

We must acknowledge that a high percentage of voice disorders are directly related to medical or organic factors and that these factors must be considered as we plan our therapy. We may feel confident, for example, that a client has vocal nodes, but this is a medical problem, and we are not qualified to make such a diagnosis. The confirmation of our clinical judgment and evaluation by a physician will justify and clarify our clinical approach to the problem. Should you seek out medical information as a standard procedure in voice therapy? We feel you should take this precaution.

Finally, with some vocal disturbances the clinician may also want to have a psychological evaluation performed. This type of evaluation may indicate that the client needs professional counseling more than he needs voice therapy or that the two services should occur in tandem. Also, keep in mind that some counseling is part of all therapy you provide. Counseling in voice therapy was discussed in detail in Chapter 5.

The voice evaluation procedures that follow are coordinated by heading and by number with the Voice Evaluation Procedures and the Voice Behavior Profile Sheet (VBPS) found in Appendix A.

GENERAL DATA GATHERING

Auditory Classification. Even though we recognize that auditory terms such as harsh or breathy are not accurate and that there is very little agreement between clinicians as to their meanings, you should auditorally classify the client's voice. It will help focus your attention on a general behavioral orientation with the client. Your choice of a term to describe the client's voice is not a critical issue as long as you are cautious when you use the term with another clinician. In that you understand what the term means, it is valid and reliable for your records. Your auditory label may include a number of terms to describe the client's voice quality, pitch, and loudness. Enter your descriptive term(s) on the Voice Behavior Profile Sheet (VBPS).

Collection of Historical Information. It is assumed that your agency has a case history form that can be modified for this step in the assessment. When taking the history, ask a series of questions about the vocal complaint. Ask what the client thinks the problem is and when it began. You should also get some information pertaining to changes in the problem over time. These questions should lead to additional questions you feel important to your data-gathering process. You are not attempting to establish a medical or psychological cause for a condition, only gathering information that might help you in deciding on a referral.

Observation of General Motor Skills. Your observations of the client's general motor activities may give you some insight into his vocal disorder. If the client has not yet been seen by a physician and you detect what you consider to be problems with motor performances, you may inform the physician of your observations so that he might more carefully evaluate this. Observe both gross and fine motor skill performances. Have the client write, walk, skip, make faces, pick up small objects off the desk, and so forth. Make notes on your observations on the VBPS.

Oral-Peripheral Examination. Perform a standard oral-peripheral examination on the client. Check the size and shape of the oral cavity, tongue, jaw, and so forth. Observe the general mobility of the oral structures. Note the size of the oropharyngeal port. It might be helpful to have the client chew, suck, and swallow so you can observe the interactions of the structures. Write your observations and findings on the VBPS.

Hearing Test. As part of your general examination procedure, you should test the client's hearing. This does not have to be an in-depth auditory analysis; a pure tone screening will do. But you do need information on the client's hearing acuity. A significant hearing loss may manifest itself in lack of or excessive vocal loudness or in the vocal quality. If you do discover some hearing loss, make a referral to an audiologist so you can obtain more complete information on the problem.

COMPETENCE/PERFORMANCE EVALUATION

Respiration

1. Breathing Patterns. Begin the assessment of specific vocal behaviors by assessing the client's breathing pattern. The proper breathing for speech is breathing that is coordinated, the abdomen and thorax moving in concert, not in opposition. During inhalation, if the abdomen moves at all, it moves outward just as the thorax does. At the same time, there is no movement of the shoulders during respiration.

In order to assess this, have the client read aloud a passage and observe his breathing pattern. Have him do this while he is standing and sitting. In addition, have him start speaking with a normal inhalation and with a deep breath. You should also carry on a conversation with him while he is standing and sitting. Note any unusual lifting of the shoulders. This is "clavicular" breathing. Also note if, when this breathing pattern occurs, opposition movement between the thorax and the abdomen is present. This is "opposition" breathing. Neither of these breathing patterns are necessarily harmful to life or to voice, but they do present the possibility that the control sought for smooth and consistent air flow will be more difficult to obtain. Next, count the number of respirations in one minute. The average individual will breathe 12 to 15 times per minute, and each cycle of respiration will appear similar. Record any unusual behaviors of respiration on the VBPS.

2. Checking Action. Checking action is the process of using muscles of inhalation during exhalation to permit release of the exhaled air stream slowly and with a constant air flow and pressure. Ask the client to take in all the air he can and then release the air (exhale) as slowly as possible. During this exhalation the client should be forming his mouth to produce a schwa vowel (but totally without sound). He should also be instructed to make certain that all his air is exhaled before stopping. You have two important tasks. The first is to time the duration of the controlled (checked) exhalation. The second is to record any difficulties or inconsistencies encountered by the client. You should obtain a minimum of three trials, recording a mean time value for the three trials. These data will be compared with other voice performance data. Both the client's mean voiceless time and behavior consistency should be recorded on the VBPS. Any score of less than 10 seconds indicates that this may be a problem area.

Phonation

Given a constant controlled air flow, two vocal behaviors are necessary for phonatory competence. The first competence is the vocal mechanism's ability to approximate the vocal folds and to maintain their approximation over time. The second competence is the vocal mechanism's ability to vibrate synchronously and maintain the synchronous vibration. The first competence, approximation, is accomplished by the intrinsic muscles of the larynx, which adduct and abduct the vocal folds. The second competence (synchrony) is determined by the comparative weight or mass of the vocal folds and is therefore an aerodynamic function.

3(a). Vocal Fold Approximation: From Open. To assess the client's ability to approximate the vocal folds, ask him to produce a series of voiceless-voiced-voiceless-voiced productions. The client may need to think about performing a slow mechanical laugh such as ha-ha-ha-ha. It is critical that during the voiceless phases of the task the air is constantly being expelled. Thus, the task is for the client to start a continuous air stream and to move the vocal folds into the position of approximation, then away from approximation, then back to approximation, and so on, while the air stream is slowly released. Several trials and demonstrations may be needed to fully evaluate this task. The client should always start with a full compliment of air and continue until all his air is expelled.

3(b). Vocal Fold Approximation: From Closed. In the second task, the client begins with a complete laryngeal stop, "opens" the vocal folds to the voicing position, returns to a stop, opens to voice, and so forth. The client can be asked to produce a rapid series of [ɑ] sounds, stopping each production fully with a laryngeal stop. Each sound production is separated from the next by a complete closure of the vocal folds.

It is important that the client be capable of producing both types of rapid laryngeal articulations. The first task, (3a), by the nature of the muscles and the magnitude of the movement, is much slower and more labored than the second, (3b). However, both are normal vocal behavioral performances and thus normal vocal competence. The voiceless-voice-voiceless task is handled by the lateral and posterior cricoarytenoid muscles, and the stop-voice-stop task is managed by the interarytenoids muscles. In terms of vocal competence, the lack of proper use of the cricoarytenoids is consistent with the occurrence of hard vocal attacks. Said another way, using the interarytenoids in start-stop voicing results in abrupt, hard vocal onset, whereas using the

—NOTES—

cricoarytenoids results in gradual, easy vocal onset. Vocal abuse clients will frequently have no difficulty with the second task but cannot perform the first. Clients with a unilateral or bilateral paralysis of the vocal folds will have difficulty performing either task.

4(a). Vocal Fold Vibration: Duration. The duration of a prolonged vocal tone provides considerable information about the mode or form of vibration of the vocal folds. We recognize that the mode of vibration of the vocal folds is not a physiological behavior; rather, it is an aerodynamic behavior. However, we still need to evaluate it. In the evaluation of checking action we asked the client to sustain a voiceless exhalation, holding the articulators in the position of the schwa vowel for as long as he could. In this task we ask the client to repeat the exercise but to vocalize the schwa vowel.

The client is asked to inhale to the maximum and then produce the longest voiced schwa vowel that he can. The duration of this effort should be measured and noted. Theoretically, the resistance to the air stream caused by the vibrating vocal folds should allow the client to produce voice time equal to or superior to his voiceless time determined in Task 2. There are two factors that might interfere with this assumption. If the vocal folds vibrate in an asynchronous form or mode, the efficiency of their closed phase is reduced and air will escape rapidly from the lungs, shortening the vocal duration time drastically. Even if the mode or form of vibration of the fold shifts back and forth between normal and asynchronous, this will also reduce the efficiency of air usage and shorten the vocal duration. If the mode of vibration is inconsistent, listen carefully to determine where and when the inconsistencies occur. Make sure that all tests are made using the same vowel, the schwa vowel. Be aware that if the client cannot effectively approximate the vocal folds (see 3a, 3b), this factor will also influence the relationship between voiced and unvoiced times.

Another way you can make a judgment of the mode or form of vibration of the vocal folds is to listen to and evaluate the quality of the voice. If the folds are vibrating in synchrony you will hear a clear tone, "normal" voice, that has clearly identifiable pitch. However, if the folds are out of synchronization, you will hear a "noise" component to the voice, usually a low pitched noise like vocal fry, a voice quality commonly described as "gravelly" or "hoarse."

4(b). Vocal Fold Vibration: Contrast. A comparable measure of the mode of vibration utilizes the [s] and [z] phonemes. Have the client produce the [s] phoneme as long as he can with a full compliment of air. After timing the [s] performance, have the client produce the [z] phoneme under the identical requirements. You have the same type of data with the [s] and [z] as you had with the voiceless and voiced schwa. You can now verify your previous result and compare the findings of sustained vowel versus sustained consonant production. The times for the two tasks should be similar for normal vocal behavior.

4(c). Vocal Fold Vibration: Stability. You should now make a judgment of the stability of the vocal fold vibrations, that is, how consistent the vibrations are over time. Your judgment is based on what you hear. Have the client talk to you. Have him relate a story, tell you about his hobby, or anything that will make him talk for a period of time. If the folds are vibrating regularly, in a synchronous mode, you will hear a clear, musical-like tone. If the folds are vibrating irregularly, you will hear "noise" mixed with the vocal tone. It is important for you to differentiate between the concepts of approximation of the vocal folds (3a, 3b), the mode of vibration of the folds (4a, 4b), and the consistency or steadiness of the vocal fold vibration. For example, a voice may be asynchronous at all times. On the other hand, a voice might be synchronous (normal tone) for a short period, lapse into asynchrony for a period, and then return to synchrony. Or the vocal folds may approximate for a short period of time (producing vocal tone) and then fail to approximate for a time (yielding aphonia). All these variations in vocal fold vibrations will be reflected in the vocal tone. The evaluation of mode of vibration involves the interaction between the anatomy, physiology, and mechanics of the vocal mechanism and the aerodynamics of the vocal airway. If there are periods of normal voice in an otherwise variable vocal production, this is a positive clinical sign. During these tasks, note the pitch and loudness levels the client elects to use to gain maximal performance (time) and the appropriateness of the vocal fold approximation (gradual or sudden) at the beginning of each task.

Laryngeal Adjustments

5(a). Pitch Level: Vocal Duration. The evaluation of pitch requires a great deal of direction and listening skill on the part of the clinician. First ask the client to take in all the air possible and sustain a tone at a pitch of his choosing until the air is gone. Time the task. Next ask the client to repeat the task at his lowest pitch. In general, low pitch voice phonation time should be slightly shorter in time than any other pitch. Now repeat the task with the client using the highest pitch he can produce. A large time discrepancy may indicate muscle control

—NOTES—

difficulty for pitch or an aerodynamic problem. You should also listen for pitch stability. Low pitch should not begin to slide upward or high pitch slide downward. Sliding is an indication of poor muscle control.

5(b). Pitch Changes: Vocal Stability. A second evaluation for pitch is pitch sliding. With a full compliment of air, have the client start at his lowest pitch and slide the pitch upward to his highest pitch. Repeat the task starting at his highest pitch and have him slide down to his lowest pitch. You should listen for missing segments of the pitch range, which is usually associated with an aerodynamic problem or unequal mass of the two vocal folds.

6(a). Loudness Level: Vocal Duration. The evaluation of vocal loudness follows the pattern established for vocal pitch. Using a full compliment of air and a pitch of the client's choosing, ask the client to sustain a schwa vowel at his choice of average loudness. Repeat the task asking the client to sustain the vowel at his softest level. Finish this section by asking the client to sustain the vowel at his loudest level. Remember that in normal voice, there is no air cost for intensity, so the times recorded should be nearly equal. Short phonation time at a soft level may indicate that the client has an approximation problem, particularly if the production lapses into aphonia or the breath stream is halted. Difficulty with time at the loudest level may indicate a lack of coordination between a constant air flow (respiration checking action) and loudness.

6(b). Loudness Change: Vocal Stability. Ask the client to inhale deeply and start at his softest voice and slowly increase loudness until he is at his loudest level, maintaining the pitch. Repeat the task from loud to soft. Listen for two common problems: First, does the client shift his loudness up or down in large units rather than in a progressive slide? This may indicate a lack of muscle control for loudness. Second, does the client modify his pitch on this task? You may need to remind him that the pitch is of his choosing but he is to maintain that pitch and change only the loudness. A failure to keep pitch constant while changing intensity may indicate that the mechanism is not behaving independently for loudness and pitch. The next section of the evaluation will verify this behavior.

7. Pitch-Loudness Interaction. The interaction between pitch and loudness is part of prosody. Prosody is the musical, contextual component of language; it includes such factors as rate, intonation, phrasing, pausing, all important factors in the oral communication process. In fact, prosody is as important to the coding and decoding of the speech message as syntax and phonology. Therefore, changes in pitch and loudness are not just a cosmetic addition to speech but rather are an important linguistic component. Clients with inadequate pitch and loudness control may lose important information in the encoding of speech. As we begin to add these components to the competence/performance evaluation, we should be aware that we are moving the client's vocal behavioral performances from simple to complex.

Since pitch and loudness are independently managed by the vocal mechanism, one important performance criterion is the independence of these two functions; that is, a normal voice should be able to change pitch without changing loudness and change loudness without changing pitch. Yet, many behavioral voice disorders demonstrate a lack of independence for pitch and loudness. For example, some clients when asked to increase loudness will also increase pitch. This lack of prosodic independence has considerable linguistic as well as vocal relevance.

To test the interactions of pitch and loudness, have the client produce the schwa vowel under the following conditions:

1. High pitch (loud voice)
2. High pitch (soft voice)
3. Low pitch (loud voice)
4. Low pitch (soft voice)
5. Low pitch ascending to high pitch (soft voice)
6. Low pitch ascending to high pitch (loud voice)
7. High pitch descending to low pitch (loud voice)
8. High pitch descending to low pitch (soft voice)
9. Soft voice increasing to loud voice (low pitch)
10. Soft voice increasing to loud voice (high pitch)
11. Loud voice descending to soft voice (high pitch)
12. Loud voice descending to soft voice (low pitch)

Observe the client carefully as he performs these tasks and make notes on his performance on the VBPS. Are pitch and loudness functioning independently, or as one changes does the other also change? Does the client have a great deal of difficulty in performing some tasks? Also, engage the client in a conversation and evaluate his prosody as he speaks. If, in your opinion, the context of the communication is impaired because of inappropriate prosody, it should be so noted on the VBPS.

Resonance Coupling

8. Nasopharyngeal Port Adjustments. The evaluation of resonance is important to our compete understanding of the aerodynamic relationships between the laryngeal system and the resonance system.

—NOTES—

Briefly, we understand that the vocal folds vibrate with an air flow from the lungs through the approximated vocal folds and up into the pharynx and oral cavity. When needed, nasal resonance is added by accessing the nasal cavity for resonance. This is accomplished by opening the nasopharyngeal port, mainly by lowering the soft palate. When nasal resonance is no longer required, the nasal cavity is isolated through closure of the nasopharyngeal port by raising the soft palate. If the isolation of the nasal cavity is not complete or if the timing of the isolation is not precise, excess nasality is heard in the voice. With the reverse, the lack of nasal resonance when it is required, the end result is the distortion of the nasalized phonemes which is usually viewed as an articulation disorder.

In order to evaluate the resonance characteristics of the client's voice, have the client count slowly from 60 to 70 on one exhalation. Velopharyngeal incompetence will be obvious during this task. The next task is designed to test the mobility of the soft palate as well as velopharyngeal competence. Have the client inhale deeply and repeat the following phonetic sequences:

1. [mpɑ/mpɑ/mpɑ/mpɑ]
2. [pɑm/pɑm/pɑm/pɑm]
3. [mɑp/mɑp/mɑp/mɑp]

Each of these tasks requires a high level of velopharyngeal mobility and timing. Normal speakers should have no vocal variations while performing these tasks. Speakers with neuromuscular coordination problems may show either voice variability or resonance assimilation. The next task is for the client to repeat each of the following syllables three times:

[im]	[mi]
[ik]	[ki]
[ih]	[hi]
[ɑm]	[mɑ]
[ɑk]	[kɑ]
[ɑh]	[hɑ]
[um]	[mu]
[uk]	[ku]
[uh]	[hu]

This combination of consonants and vowels gives a good overview of the mobility and coordination of the soft palate. Note any difficulties the client may have with this task. The final task for the client is to speak while using an exaggerated jaw opening. The lack of opening the mouth while speaking may be contributing to excessive nasal resonance. Any disturbances in the resonance balance of the voice should be noted on the VBPS.

INTEGRATED VOCAL ANALYSIS

In this assessment you will be considering the end product of all the behavioral performances you just evaluated: the client's voice production. Yes, we still depend on some subjective appraisals. There are neither instruments nor adequate normative data to substitute for the trained ear of the clinician. You must determine if the client has a voice problem and, if so, in what aspect of vocal production. You are now doing an auditory analysis, indicating where problems exist so you can focus your therapy on the particular behavioral deficit. Keep in mind that sometimes a person can perform a behavior in isolation but not when integrated into other behaviors, such as producing a correct phoneme in isolation but not in ongoing speech. Conversely, and especially in vocal behaviors, it is not unusual for a client to be unable to adequately perform a behavior in isolation but able to perform it satisfactorily in ongoing speech. This is because most people have very little voluntary control over their laryngeal activities. The laryngeal changes and adjustments that do occur are more reflexive and involuntary than voluntary. If asked to close their vocal folds these people would not know how to accomplish the task. However, if they were asked to hold their breath, they would have no difficulty in performing the task.

There will not be perfect agreement between your findings on the conpetence/performance evaluation and this assessment. However, in the main, this assessment is a confirmation of the findings in the evaluation. You must have the client speak for an extended period of time. You can have him tell a story, explain a hobby, or tell about anything else that will necessitate his doing most of the talking during the evaluation. You will be listening and observing, gathering data in order to make some decisions. You will evaluate each of the following factors in terms of its function in the overall speech of the client:

1. *Breathing patterns.* If the client manifests no breathing difficulties during his speech, you will make no mark on the form. However, if you observe opposition breathing or clavicular breathing that appears to interfere with the client's speech, indicate a breathing problem by entering a *Bp*– in the appropriate cell.

—NOTES—

2. *Checking action*. You will ignore this factor if the client manifests no difficulty in maintaining appropriate phrasing and speech loudness over time. If the client does have difficulty in this area, enter a *Ca–* on the form.

3. *Vocal fold approximation*. You will be listening for voice quality, which indicates that the vocal fold approximation is either inadequate or excessive. If the voice sounds as though the approximation is inadequate and you can hear air escaping, the voice is "breathy"; mark *Ai* on the form. If the voice indicates that the approximation is excessive and you can hear vocal strain, the voice is "choked"; mark *Ae* on the form. It is also very important for you to listen for excessive use of the hard vocal onset, that is, the client initiating vocalization from the closed position of the vocal folds so that voicing is introduced very abruptly. This is a relatively common vocal behavior but when used excessively it can cause vocal irritation. If this is present, note this on the form and enter an *Ho*. Finally, if there are indications that the vocal fold approximation varies during speech (the voice varies spasmodically between being "breathy" and "choked") mark *Av* on the form.

4. *Vocal fold mode of vibration*. As was mentioned earlier, this is an aerodynamic behavior of the vocal folds, not a physiological one. However, the mode of vibration of the vocal folds is a vital factor in vocal quality. If the vocal folds are vibrating in a regular, synchronous mode, you will hear normal voice quality, clear of noise factors. In this event, leave the cell empty. However, if the vocal folds are asynchronous in their vibrations, each fold vibrating at a different frequency (you will hear noise in the vocal tone), the voice is "hoarse," and you should enter an *S–* on the form. If the mode of vibration shifts back and forth from synchronous to asynchronous, enter an *Sv* on the form.

5. *Pitch level*. The correct pitch of a voice is related to the physiology of the larynx. Correct pitch appears to be about four or five musical tones above the lowest note the person can sing. Your task here is to determine if the client's general vocal pitch is, in your opinion, appropriate for his age and size. You already have the data on his pitch range so you have some idea of where his pitch should be. If there is not an apparent problem, leave the cell empty. However, if the vocal pitch is a problem, enter a *P+* on the form if it is too high or a *P–* if the pitch is too low.

6. *Loudness level*. The loudness of the voice is a very subjective assessment and can, in many instances, be a reflection of the personality of the client. Again, you have data concerning the client's

loudness range so you know how loud or soft he can speak. You now must judge if you think he is speaking at an appropriate loudness level for the situation he is in. If there is no apparent problem, leave the cell empty. But if the vocal loudness is a problem, enter an $L+$ for a voice that is too loud or an $L-$ for a voice that is too soft.

7. *Prosody*. You are now concerned with the interaction of pitch and loudness as they convey the context of the vocal message. You will not be concerned with inappropriate melody, rhythm, and accent that is associated with dialectal or regional speech. Your concern here is with the range of pitch and loudness interaction. If there is no apparent problem with prosody, leave the cell empty. However, if you hear speech that would be labeled monotone, enter a $Pr-$ on the form. Conversely, if the variations in pitch and loudness are excessive, constituting prosody that might be associated with an athetoid child, enter a $Pr+$ on the form.

8. *Nasal resonance*. You are now judging the amount and the type of nasality present in the client's speech. When considering the amount of nasality, excessive nasal resonance in the speech should be rated $N+$ on the form while insufficient nasality should be rated $N-$.

ENVIRONMENTAL GUIDANCE OF VOCAL BEHAVIORS

The final step in the voice evaluation assesses the influence on vocal production by changes in the client's internal and external environment. These manipulations of the environment often bring about perceptible changes in voice production. If these environmental changes provoke positive changes in vocal production, they can be used as clinical strategies in the client's therapy.

The first task calls for the client to speak to the clinician as the distance between them is increased. The client is instructed to use a voice that is just loud enough to "reach" the clinician. Note the client's ability to maintain vocal integrity as he speaks louder. The second task calls for the client to speak over and under a "barrier." In this task, raise a sheet of paper or a book about 2 feet over your head and ask the client to face straight ahead but to "project" his voice *over* the barrier. Listen carefully for vocal changes. Next lower the barrier to 1 foot off the ground and ask the client to "project" his voice *under* the barrier. We are not certain how these visual projection aids work, but clients frequently produce a better or a worse voice under these conditions.

The final tasks examine vocal production during changes in the internal environment, that is, in the body. You will be concerned with vocal changes that occur with increased body tension, during relaxation, and with changes in spatial relationships associated with the larynx. The test of vocal production under tension may be achieved by asking the client to tighten all the muscles in his body, hold this state for 5 seconds, and then produce a long sustained schwa vowel. You might have him attempt to lift the chair he is seated on by pulling up on the seat. In order to evaluate the effects of relaxation, you may need to use the relaxation techniques found in Appendix B. When the client is noticeably more relaxed, have him produce the long sustained schwa vowel. Note differences in production between a schwa vowel produced under tension and one produced while more relaxed.

The final task consists of having the client continuously vocalize a vowel as he slowly lowers his head until his chin is resting on his chest. Then reverse the process and have the client vocalize as he raises his head back to the normal position. Note any changes in vocal production. Now repeat the procedure but have the client slowly raise his head until he is looking at the ceiling over his head. Then repeat as he lowers his head to the normal position. Again note changes in vocal production. Differences in vocal performances in any of these tasks are indicators of probable etiology and are important for therapy planning, particularly if the environmental guidance given to the client results in improved vocal performance.

RESULTS OF THE EVALUATION

Having collected all of your data, you are now ready to make some very important decisions. Your first decision concerns whether or not your client has a handicapping vocal disorder. Your decision will be based on the attitudes and feelings of the client, the data collected, the policies of your agency, and your professional opinion. There are no absolutes here; you can only depend on yourself as a professional. If you have serious doubts, ask a colleague to assist you. Everyone enjoys having his opinion asked for and advice is cheap. You do not have to follow the advice, just receive it.

Before we get much further we must compare the data collected in the voice evaluation. We are dealing with four possible conditions when we compare the findings of the competence/performance evaluation and the data from the VBPS. Obviously, if the client performs normally on both evaluations, there is no clinical problem. If the client fails the same general items on both evaluations, you can feel very secure when planning therapy that the behaviors in question are truly problematic. Your therapy should start with the first behavior in the sequence whose performance is not adequate. You start with the most basic behavior and build up from it, building voice from the breath support foundation to the final touches of resonance. However, it is important to recognize that if the client has failed to perform a given behavior on both evaluations, you will be, in essence, teaching the client to perform a new behavior that does not exist in his vocal behavioral repertoire.

Now, let us consider conflicts between the competence/performance evaluation and the integrated voice analysis. Let us consider a client who fails some of the competence tests but whose integrated voice analysis is normal. Consider the reflexive-involuntary nature of the larynx and you can understand how a client might not be able to perform a task on a voluntary level but can then perform it normally on a reflexive speech level. If there are no indications of behavioral disruption of voice on the voice analysis, dismiss the client: He has no vocal problems.

Let us now reverse the problem—you have a client who performs the tasks in the competence/performance evaluation correctly but whose voice analysis indicates that there are behaviors that are interfering with normal vocal production. You could plan your therapy based on the performance on the voice analysis as you did earlier but this time you would know that the client is able to perform the tasks in isolation or in special circumstances. This would be akin to a client performing correctly on an articulation test but displaying articulation errors in his ongoing speech, not an unheard of situation. However, because the client was able to perform the behaviors normally on the evaluation is a positive clinical sign, indicating that the behavior does exist in the client's behavioral repertoire, just not in ongoing speech. You will not be teaching him a new behavior, just a new place to perform an existing behavior.

If, after considering all factors, you have concluded that the client does indeed have a handicapping vocal disorder and that therapy is indicated, you must now determine which behaviors are contributing to the vocal problem and why the behaviors are not being performed satisfactorily. You may not be able to determine the reasons for faulty behavioral performance (etiology) until you receive additional information from other professionals. This is the reason for referrals, to determine medical or psychological causes, or to eliminate them as possibilities. How important is it to establish a cause? It is crucial! You can only

—NOTES—

plan effective and efficient therapy if it is planned with an etiological factor in mind. And what do you do if there is no medical or psychological explanation for a problem behavior? You must assume it is a learned behavior and, with this etiological factor in mind, plan your therapy accordingly.

It is extremely important to remember that, in behavior therapy, voice therapy is not different from articulation therapy. In both cases you are interested in modifying a behavior that has been interfering with his communication. If the client has a medical problem such as a paralyzed tongue or vocal fold, we still modify the behavior but we set up a different behavior change goal, one that accepts less then perfect performance. If an emotional problem exists, we decide if we can deal with it in therapy or if we should refer the client. Medical, organic, and psychological factors are only intervening variables that we must try to work around, planning our therapy in such a way that the factor has a minimal influence on the treatment procedure.

Before we move into the clinical process, let us consider how we work with the physician in the event there is a pathologic condition involved in the vocal disorder. We are primarily interested in avoiding anything in therapy that would aggravate the medical condition. In other words, if the condition is due to laryngeal tension, we would not want to include any strategies that would increase laryngeal tension. Further, in order to know what effect therapy is having on the vocal folds, we must have the physician do periodic checks to determine their condition. His reports will tell us if we are making progress in eliminating factors that are abusing the folds. There is one other situation to consider before moving on. If you are convinced the vocal disorder is due to a medical problem such as vocal nodes but the examining physician reports no pathologic change, you should seek a second opinion. Physicians, just like speech clinicians, sometimes err.

You are now ready to start planning your therapy. Establish your behavior change goals based on the information contained in the VBPS. If the client could not perform the target behavior in either evaluation condition, plan to teach the behavior as a new behavior. If the behavior already exists in isolation, you must now get the behavior to occur in context with speech. Plan your therapy around the guidelines presented in the chapter dealing with cognitive behavior therapy.

Chapter 7

The Clinical Conference

THE SCHOOL ENVIRONMENT

Because of a variety of federal, state, and district regulations, your clinical interactions with clients in the school environment are carefully structured. We will assume that you have received permission to evaluate the client and have, after gathering all the necessary data, planned your treatment program for the client. The most crucial part of the process is the Individual Educational Planning Conference (IEPC), since it is here that the decision is made as to whether or not the client may receive therapy.

As you prepare to discuss the evaluation and recommendations with parents, keep in mind who referred the client for the evaluation. If the parents were involved in this action, you can assume some interest and motivation on their part. However, if you initiated the action and they have only been passively involved in the procedure, recognize their probable lack of motivation to have their child receive therapy.

When you discuss your findings with the parents in the IEPC, it is important to remember that the parents do not understand the complexities of vocal production and vocal disorders. In some instances, depending on the severity of the vocal problem, the parents will also be emotionally involved with the problem. Avoid the use of professional jargon, particularly anatomical and physiological terms; use terms that the parent will understand.

One of the most difficult factors you may have to deal with is to convince the parents that their child actually does have a vocal problem. If the problem might lead to a medical condition, such as incorrect vocal behaviors leading to vocal nodes, you may have an easier chance of convincing the parents that therapy is called for. However, as was pointed out in the first chapter, society is not all that concerned about voices that "deviate." Because you have gone this far in the clinical process, having an IEPC, we can assume that you feel that therapy is strongly indicated for this client. Prepare your presentation carefully, since, in the event the parents are not concerned about the child's voice, you will have to convince them of the seriousness of the problem.

You should make sure that the parents have a basic understanding of the voice problem and how you plan to treat it. Explain carefully what vocal behaviors you are going to change and why they need to be changed. Then, set your therapy program forth in distinct stages, that is, getting the new behavior to occur, stabilizing it, and generalizing the new behavior to all speaking environments. Explain how you will achieve each of these clinical goals. If your program will include a home program to supplement your therapy, explain this carefully to the parents. Be specific in terms of how much time you want them to spend with the home program and how you will work with them. This might be extremely important with very young clients. If the parents agree that their child may receive therapy, you should get as much information from them as possible to assist you with your therapy.

AREAS TO EXPLORE WITH PARENTS

1. You should determine the parents' feelings as to why their child has the voice problem. This may be the source of some anxiety in the home and even negative reactions to the child.
2. Ask the parents how they respond to their child's voice in the home. They can only respond one of three ways: They can reward the child by being solicitous, penalize the child by a negative reaction, or ignore the child's voice by not reacting to it.
3. Another important area of questioning concerns the reactions of siblings to the child's voice. Your questions should include both younger and older siblings.
4. Playmates are a peer group for the child, and you should discuss with the parents how playmates react to the child's voice.
5. The home environment should be carefully examined. Is the home environment quiet and unhurried or are there numerous activities taking place and a high level of noise? Does the child have to talk over others to get people's attention? This will call for some subtle questions.
6. If you do plan to have a home program to supplement your direct therapy with the client, inquire about the willingness of the parents to carry on a home program. Again, carefully set forth what you expect the parents to do, why they would be doing it, how often they should do it, and how long each home session might last. Do

not be surprised if the parents agree to work with you but then fail to follow through. At this time you are only interested in the parents' initial response to your request for assistance. The follow-through, or lack of, will have to be dealt with later in your therapy.

MINI-REFERENCE FOR PUBLIC LAW 92-142

For your convenience, an overview of Public Law (PL) 92-142 is presented here. This is an excerpt from "A Mini-manual for Teachers in Special Education Programs" by Dr. Mae Taylor, Specialist in Communication Disorders, Utah State Office of Education. This is not meant to be a replacement or substitute for the more detailed federal document nor for local or state interpretation; it is meant only as a handy reference for the clinician and is an example of one state's document to assist personnel in programs for the handicapped in the schools.

PERMISSION FOR TESTING/EVALUATION

1. Permission for testing forms must include the following: (1) areas in which tests are to be administered; (2) names and purpose of the tests in each area; (3) date; (4) signature of the person sending the form to the parents; (5) the reason(s) for testing. All of the above items must be completed prior to sending the form to the parents for their signature.
2. Permission by a parent must be given by a signed and dated signature. If there are boxes, which are to be checked for indicating permission or refusal, included on the form, the appropriate box must be clearly checked.
3. Permission for testing shall never post date the *actual* testing date.
4. Permission for testing needs to be re-obtained only if it is determined that areas will be tested for which existing permission is not now granted.

DIAGNOSIS AND ASSESSMENT

1. Diagnostic protocols, or summary reports, must be included in a student's folder in order to support the student's classification of handicapping condition.
2. More than one measure must be used to determine classification or handicapping condition. (In the case of an articulation disorder the two measures might be (1) a standardized test of articulation and (2) observation of the student's articulation in conversational speech).
3. Protocols and reports must be signed in full and dated as to day, month, and year.

4. Testing instruments must be selected so as to measure the student's natural ability and not reflect environmental, sensory (visual or auditory), physical, or ethnic background.
5. Classification must be made by a multi-disciplinary team or group of persons.

INDIVIDUALIZED EDUCATION PROGRAM (IEP)

1. Completion of blanks: All sections and spaces contained on the district's/agency's IEP form must be completed (filled in), including: (1) the student's classifying information; (2) the student's present levels of achievement; (3) strengths; (4) weaknesses; (5) annual goals; (6) short-term objectives which are measurable.
2. Signatures: The team's complete signatures must be individually dated in full (day, month, year).
3. Classification: Classification must be written out, as opposed to initialed or coded, on the IEP, and fully explained to the parents.
4. Focus on the learning problem: Annual goals and short-term objectives must be focused on the student's problem.
5. Review: IEP must be reviewed and updated as often as required, but *at least annually.*

PARTICIPANTS IN MEETINGS

1. All IEP meetings conducted for all categories of handicapping conditions must utilize the minimum number of participants: (1) local district or agency representative; (2) the student's teacher; (3) the parent or guardian.

PERMISSION FOR PLACEMENT

1. The IEP spells out or dictates the placement of the student.
2. The IEP must be fully completed *before* placement occurs (services begin).
3. All required information on the Permission to Place form must be completed including: (1) description of placement options considered; (2) reason(s) for proposed placement including the anticipated length of service; (3) name, date and title of the the person completing the form; (4) parental permission must be clearly indicated and signed in full including the date of the signature; (5) other alternatives considered and rejected are no longer mandatory, but remain a good practice.
4. A new Permission for Placement form does not need to be re-obtained unless the student's placement option is changed.
5. The permission for placement form must be signed by the parent *before* the student can be serviced.

TERMINATION

1. When it is determined that a student can be released from special education services, the action must be accomplished through the IEP process. The same kind of meeting held to classify the student and write the IEP must be held to declassify.
2. When students move from school to school, or between levels (elementary to junior high to senior high), they are still classified as handicapped unless a declassification meeting is held. If they are not declassified, they must be served. A move between levels is not justification for terminating special education services to the student.
3. When the parents or students refuse the services offered, the agency is strongly advised to provide a form for parents to sign indicating that services have been offered but refused.

OTHER REQUIRED DOCUMENTATION

Location of documentations listed may vary, depending upon state or district practices.

1. Primary language of the home: The primary language needs to be documented in the student's folder and is frequently placed on the IEP form.
2. Justification for Placement: A justification for the placement option selected is most often found on the IEP form. Options considered must be listed on the Permission for Placement form.
3. Due Process Information Dissemination: Documentation of dissemination of due process information (rights of parents) must be presented.
4. Record of Access: A Record of Access form must be available for use before a student's file is accessed.
5. Access and Authorization: A file access authorization list shall be maintained for public inspection and shall include a full listing of the names and positions of those staff members who may have access to personally indentifiable information. The list shall be updated as necessary and shall include the following six categories: (1) name of staff member who has permission to access the records; (2) position of staff member who may access records; (3) name of the district; (4) name of the school; (5) school year in which effective; (6) identification of records manager.
6. Services Mandatory: Any student classified as handicapped for educational purposes must be served—there can be no waiting list.

Section III
The Therapy Process

Chapter 8

Factors Influencing Therapy

INTERVENING FACTORS THAT INTERFERE WITH THERAPY

As we begin our discussion of treatment of voice disorders, it is very important that we recognize that in some instances, because of an intervening organic or psychological factor, vocal behaviors are not performed or they are performed inadequately. When such a factor is present, it influences our therapy in that it forces us to adapt our therapy to the interfering factor. Often, the factor also affects the effectiveness and efficiency of our therapy. So before we get too deeply into our therapy approaches to the various behavioral deficiencies, let us consider what those factors are and how they might interfere with our treatment program and goals.

Organic Problems

There are a number of organic problems that can interfere with behavioral performances. Without going into detail we should consider structural deviations resulting from fractures or developmental problems. Another source of structural deviation is growths on the vocal folds such as vocal nodes or polyps. There are also neurological problems that interfere with laryngeal behavioral performance. Of course, there are also a number of diseases of the larynx that interfere with behavioral performances. We will attempt to discuss the most common problems as we present the therapy program for the various vocal behaviors.

When we encounter organic problems associated with a vocal disorder, we must determine if the organic factor is reversible, such as with vocal nodes, or irreversible, as in the case of laryngeal paralysis. This information can be provided by the physician who examines the client.

If the condition is due to inappropriate vocal habits and is reversible, our goal of therapy should be to eliminate the abusive vocal be-

—NOTES—

haviors and see if this, in turn, eliminates the organic factor. We may find that there is no need for further voice therapy. For example, if the vocal behavior of proper approximation of the vocal folds is interfered with by vocal nodes, our therapy should be designed to remove the vocal abusive behaviors that caused the nodes to form. If our treatment program is effective and the nodes are absorbed, chances are that the vocal fold approximation behavior will occur naturally and the vocal disorder will no longer exist. It is very important for us to know whether or not an organic factor that is interfering with our therapy can be reversed. We cannot plan appropriate therapy without this information since it determines our clinical goal.

If the condition is irreversible, as with the laryngeal paralysis, we must adjust our clinical goal accordingly. We cannot achieve the goal of a normal voice if a required behavior cannot be performed. In this instance we may not establish a firm clinical goal, since we do not know how closely the client can approximate normal vocal production. We re-evaluate our clinical goal according to the progress we are making in therapy. Our clinical goal is then flexible, determined by how much progress we can make in therapy.

An organic problem we must also consider is hearing impairment. Not only are we dependent on the client's auditory perception of the disorder in order to correct it but the hearing problem may be the cause of the disorder. A hearing problem certainly could be involved in a loudness problem and might also be involved in pitch and quality problems. This factor should be assessed during any voice evaluation.

Functional Problems

In addition to structural factors, we must also be aware of functional factors that can create clinical problems. Emotional factors such as hysterical conversion responses can negate our therapy. Emotional stress can also influence the vocal performance of clients and interfere with our treatment program. In addition, perhaps one step beyond stress, is the conditioned emotional response to certain talking situations. A conditioned emotional response to a speaking situation can inhibit the performance of certain vocal behaviors and thus create voice problems. In this situation, therapy must be aimed at changing the conditioned response, since this is the reason the behavior is not being performed.

If the vocal disorder is directly related to an emotional problem, such as with hysterical aphonia, professional counseling is indicated.

Direct therapy on the vocal disorder will be of no avail, because the disorder will be maintained by the emotional conflict. However, even if the emotional problem is resolved, the client may still manifest a vocal problem, perhaps due to vocal abuse that resulted from the emotional conflict. So even though a client may be referred for counseling, there should be a follow-up exam to make sure that the vocal problem was dealt with in the counseling.

BASELINE DATA

All therapy has a focus and our therapy focuses on the level of competence of the behavior we are going to modify in therapy; that is, we take the existing proficiency of the behavior and use this as a base to compare all future performances. If the performance of the behavior improves, we can then assume our therapy is being effective. Conversely, if the behavioral performance does not improve, we must review our treatment plan. We turn back to the CIM model in Figure 2; it provides a means of resolving the problem.

We have two types of data that we can use to judge the progress of our therapy, the data we collected on the competence/performance evaluation and the data on the integrated voice analysis. These data provide us with a baseline, the level of performance of the client when we first evaluated his voice. We now have two ways to evaluate the effectiveness of our therapy, a cross-check, if you will.

You should periodically test the client's performance on the tasks involved in the competence/performance evaluation. Compare his current performance levels with his performance during the evaluation. Is the duration of prolonged tones longer? Is he better able to produce vocal fold opening and closing procedures? Is he able to produce pitch changes without changing loudness levels? This information will give you a good appraisal of the effectiveness of your therapy.

The second clinical check is the integrated vocal analysis we performed as part of the voice evaluation. We rated the client on the presence of problematic vocal behaviors and how these behaviors influenced the voice. We rated the adequacy of vocal behaviors as performed in on-going speech. You should perform this analysis periodically to see if there has been a change in the overall voicing of the client.

CLINICAL STRATEGIES

The clinical strategies used with all voice clients are all based on the CIM model. Rather than restrict you to a specific list of clinical techniques, we present you with the ingredients, the basic concepts involved, and allow you to create your own clinical technique. In this way, your only limitation is your imagination. Let us quickly review the basic strategies you have at your disposal.

Modeling

Modeling behaviors is a quick and simple means to convey behavioral information to the client. Modeling is always accompanied with some behavioral information or verbal guidance. There are two basic forms of modeling, presenting visual or auditory models. When the clinician demonstrates the desired behavior for the client, she is not only showing him how to perform the desired behavior but also making the behavior change goal clear to him. However, there are some drawbacks to modeling when it is applied to voice therapy. For example, if you are teaching easy vocal onset and want to use modeling, it means that you must be able to perform the behavior. If you cannot perform a behavior, you cannot use modeling.

A second problem with modeling is that some behaviors, such as easy vocal onset, cannot be observed by the client. This does not mean you cannot use modeling, just that you must recognize that your model is an auditory one, one that does not give basic behavioral information but only the auditory by-product of the behavioral performance. This is much more abstract, more cognitive, than the observable model.

Guidance

Guidance can occur either during our presentation of the stimulus to the client or during his response to our stimulus. Furthermore, there are four distinct forms of guidance we can use in therapy.

Gestural Guidance. Gestural guidance is any movement we make to cue or prompt a behavior to occur. This may be a body movement, a hand gesture, a facial expression, or any other type of movement. It can occur as part of our stimulus, such as a hand gesture indicating a high pitch as we model the pitch level, or it can occur as the client is responding to our stimulus, the gesture occurring as the client is attempting to produce a high pitch.

Physical Guidance. Anytime we touch the client in an attempt to assist him in performing a behavior, we are providing physical guidance. Again, it can occur during either our stimulus or the client's response. If a clinician is trying to achieve relaxation in a client's strap muscles prior to his attempting to produce vocalization and she massages his neck, this is physical guidance.

Verbal Guidance. Verbal guidance consists of cues or prompts we use to assist the client to produce a behavior. As with all other forms of guidance, it can occur either during the presentation of our stimulus or as the client is responding. It is not behavioral information as much as it is a hint or clue for the client. For example, if we are working with a client to lower his pitch, we might ask him to talk at his new pitch level and then add, "Remember, talk low, low, low." As the client is responding we might say to him, "Lower, lower." We are now providing him with verbal guidance as he is responding.

Environmental Guidance. We use environmental guidance when we want the client to respond "spontaneously," that is, without a model or obvious prompt. An example of the use of environmental guidance would involve a client whose clinical problem was speech that was too soft but who can increase his loudness to normal levels when requested. In order to provide environmental guidance we might have a radio playing when the client came in for therapy. The radio would be on loud enough to necessitate talking slightly louder to be heard over it. We would carefully not adjust our loudness level to the ambient noise (no model) but would wait to see if the client would perform his new behavior when it was appropriate.

Information

Information flows two ways in any clinical interaction. You not only provide information for the client but also request information from the client. Your entire history-taking procedure is based on your asking for information, and your therapy is often influenced by your client's opinions about his disorder or the form or direction he feels his therapy should take.

There are two basic forms of information, behavioral and general. Behavioral information takes several forms. We can give information on how to perform a behavior, such as telling a client to make a small [h] sound before saying a word and in this way getting the easy vocal onset to occur. Behavioral information might also consist of telling a client the consequences of vocal abuse or how to avoid vocal abuse.

We use behavioral information whenever we tell a client something about his vocal behavior. General information is the rest of the information we give the client in the clinical situation. This is interaction with the client that is more general in nature, such as making the next appointment or giving a homework assignment.

Shaping

In its purest form, shaping is an extremely inefficient system for teaching a new behavior. Its inefficiency is primarily due to the lack of direction provided in shaping; that is, the behavior change goal is not established for the individual. The only way the new behavior is achieved is through rewards provided to behaviors that approximate the desired behavior, a process known as "successive approximation." For example, if you want to train your dog to sit in the corner, you start by rewarding the dog each time it faces the corner, then rewarding the dog when it moves toward the corner, and so forth. It would be much simpler if you could just show the dog what you wanted by modeling the sitting behavior. But most dogs would not have the cognitive ability to recognize this as the behavioral goal; they would just think you were acting very strange, sitting in the corner. With animals with "limited" cognitive ability, you must go through the entire shaping process.

However, we work with humans, and humans have the cognitive ability to understand a behavioral goal if we tell them what it is or show it to them. Thus, we provide the client with a stimulus that sets forth the behavioral goal. We usually model the behavior and explain it. This increases the efficiency of the shaping process, since the client then not only knows the specific goal behavior he is trying to produce but also has had it explained and demonstrated.

Another way we increase the efficiency of the shaping process is to introduce penalty. We penalize those behaviors that do not approximate the behavioral goal. In pure shaping these behaviors are "ignored," that is, they have no contingent event, and hypothetically this should lead to the extinction of the incorrect behaviors. Indeed, this may eventually occur. However, in our teaching mode we cannot wait for time to take its toll on the incorrect behavior. Rather, we penalize it, reducing its frequency of occurrence, and then substitute the new, correct behavior for it.

A client may be able to speak at two pitch levels, the correct and the incorrect levels. As we penalize the incorrect one, its occurrence is reduced and it is replaced with the correct level. When the correct level occurs, it is rewarded, which increases its frequency of occurrence.

The shaping process used in this clinical approach, then, is modified in several ways to increase its efficiency. First, we provide our clients with the behavioral change goal of therapy. We also provide feedback for the client in the form of penalty for incorrect behavioral performances. With these additions, it is a very effective and efficient clinical teaching process.

The Token Economy

The token economy is a specialized system of dispensing rewards and applying penalties to a client. It is unique in that the initial reward is only a symbolic reward that can be turned in later for a meaningful reward. Our monetary system is an example of a token economy. We work and are paid for our work with tokens—money. We then use our money to purchase meaningful rewards such as food and shelter. The token economy is no more than the application of these principles to the clinic room. When the client "works" and produces the new speech behavior, he is "paid" for it, perhaps given a poker chip or some other form of token. Over a series of productions he gathers enough tokens to "purchase" something that he wants. This is called a back-up reward. The clinician has a "store" that consists of a box or a case containing a number of different items that a client might "purchase." Each item is marked as to its "cost," and the client is allowed to buy the thing he wants the most and that he can afford. The clinician's store is opened according to the way she set up her economy with the client or clients. But the store should be opened often enough so that the clients continue to be motivated to receive the tokens for the store.

The advantages of this kind of reward system are that the system provides a single reward for all clients in a group (the token); the rewards are simple to administer; and it provides a variety of back-up rewards so each client can chose the reward he wants, which makes the reward very strong. This is a powerful teaching and learning tool, and once you are familiar with its easy and flexible operation, you will find it a valuable technique.

GROUP OR INDIVIDUAL THERAPY?

Given the choice, would you prefer individual or group therapy for your clients? Before you answer the question, perhaps you should consider which stage of therapy the clients are in. Perhaps individual therapy is more suited for the first stage of therapy, since the first stage involves a great deal of individualized teaching. In this instance, you need tight control over the learning environment and the client in order for efficient learning to take place. Therefore, for those clients who are just learning their new behaviors, individual therapy would probably be the most effective and efficient.

As you move into the second stage of therapy, stabilizing the new behavior in the clinical environment, there are some other clinical issues to consider before making a choice. Because the behavior has already been learned, intense teaching interaction is no longer necessary. You are now stabilizing the behavioral performance and "generalizing" it into other speech behaviors in the clinical environment. It is here that, for a young man whose voice pitch has changed dramatically under your direction, he must learn to use the new pitch while speaking on any topic and to any person in his environment. The clinical environment is very restricted when you are providing individual therapy. You are the only person interacting with your client. However, if the client were in group therapy, these limitations would not be imposed and your therapy would be more beneficial to your client. So, perhaps at this stage of therapy, group therapy would be the therapy mode of choice.

In the final stage of therapy, generalizing the new behaviors to speaking environments outside the clinic room, you will also find that individual therapy is more limiting than group therapy. At this stage of therapy the client is reporting his success (or failure) at using the new speech behavior outside therapy. He now needs support for his efforts: rewards for his success in generalizing his new behavior. What better source of rewards than his peers in a group? In the event he has failures to report, who could understand better and provide more moral support than his peers? This is his support system.

If you have the option of selecting either group or individual therapy, consider the strong and weak points of each at different points in therapy. If you opt for group therapy, the shaping group is discussed in detail in Chapter 4.

CLIENT MOTIVATION

We should not assume that all our clients, even though they have a voice disorder, are interested in receiving voice therapy. Although some clients may seek help for their voice problem, most are sent to us for therapy. Regardless of why the client comes for assistance, the effectiveness of our therapy is directly related to the client's motivation. If a client comes to us for help, we can assume that there is some approach motivation and by using appropriate rewards in our therapy we can strengthen or maintain the motivation.

But how do we deal with the client who is *sent* to us for therapy? With no motivation for therapy we must create "artificial" approach motivation through our rewards. If our rewards are appropriate and strong, we can create approach motivation in the therapy environment. However, we will have to make further adjustments in our treatment program when it is time to generalize the new vocal behaviors to environments where we no longer have direct control over the rewards. Since we face a unique clinical situation with each type of client, we will discuss each of these conditions, motivated clients and unmotivated clients, and consider the clinical influence of the client's attitude toward therapy.

Clients Seeking Therapy

With the client seeking therapy, the existing approach motivation must be maintained. This is achieved through the clinical rewards he receives. However, as the new vocal behavior becomes more generalized and the speech more "normal," approach motivation wanes. The vocal disorder is no longer a problem, it is now just an annoyance, and as such does not demand a high priority. At this time, in order to maintain the motivation of the client, we must find a reward that will create artificial approach motivation or, perhaps, find a penalty that the client wants to avoid and thus create avoidance motivation. This provides us with two forms of motivation to use with the client.

We can also use the influence of the client's significant others, especially the parents of younger clients, to help maintain the approach and avoidance motivation. However, this depends on their availability and cooperation. If the significant others are not available or cooperative, we must turn to different means to maintain the motivation. Let us consider the two alternatives.

Cooperative Significant Others. With significant others who are cooperative, we can create a "support system." A support system consists of significant others who understand why the client is in therapy and support his efforts to modify his vocal disorder. They provide both incentives and rewards for the client as well as moral support during his therapy. This calls for counseling the significant others in terms of what and when to reward and how to support the client. This type of assistance will increase the efficiency of our therapy.

Uncooperative or Absent Significant Others. The task of strengthening or maintaining the approach motivation is now more difficult since the clinician and the client are the only people involved. There is no outside support system. In order to compensate for this we can attempt to enlist the assistance of other people in the client's environment, such as teachers, counselors, or other people in the school environment. If these people will provide understanding and support, the task of maintaining the motivation is easier. The rewards the client receives from these people are very important, since they supplement the rewards that the client is receiving from us in therapy. If this type of support program is set up, you must coordinate it if it is to be consistent.

Clients Sent for Therapy

These are the clients whose parents or teachers recommend therapy. Usually, these clients do not see any reason for changing their voice. Regardless of the reasons for their reluctance to enter therapy, it still means that they have no motivation to work on their voice. We have problems in dealing with the unmotivated client. Our task is to create motivation, since without it, our therapy will have little effect. We may have limited success creating motivation by discussing the problem with the client, but in the main, this can be used only with older and more mature clients. In this highly cognitive approach we can discuss the problems that the client faces and how therapy can help, such as with the elimination of vocal abuse. Discussions can be an important part of creating motivation, but this must be supplemented with rewards that create approach motivation. The approach motivation we create this way may be artificial, but as long as the client learns new vocal behaviors, the reason he is learning is not important.

Again, as the new vocal behaviors become more effective and the voice disorder becomes less of a problem, the approach motivation may fade. We may have to turn to avoidance motivation to maintain interest in therapy.

Cooperative Significant Others. With cooperative significant others we can create a strong "support system" that will create some motivation in the client. Their reward program can provide us with valuable assistance as we attempt to motivate the client for therapy. The significant others must be carefully counseled in this situation. They must understand that the client has no interest in therapy but that their special assistance will help motivate the client. The significant other's reward program should be carefully supervised through reports and conferences. You must be aware of what is happening with the client in the significant other's environment.

Uncooperative or Absent Significant Others. Unfortunately, this is probably the most common and the most difficult clinical task we face. We are attempting to do therapy with a client who does not want to be in therapy and whose significant others cannot or will not help us. Artificial approach motivation can be created in the clinical environment through our rewards, but once the client leaves this environment, there is no one to maintain the motivation. We can again turn to the assistance of teachers, counselors, and others in the school environment; however, this only partially replaces the support system that the client needs. This program must be carefully supervised so that it has consistency. This clinical situation is not hopeless, but our clinical skills are taxed to the utmost to motivate the client for therapy. This is not an ideal clinical situation and it does not allow us to provide the most effective therapy for the client. However, it is a common enough clinical situation that we learn to cope with it the best we can. This is the true test of all of our clinical skills.

PEER PRESSURE

Peer pressure is a factor faced in the schools, regardless of the age of the client; the pressure appears in different forms between the early elementary ages and the late high school ages. It is probably at its peak somewhere between seventh and tenth grade, depending on the individual child. Peer pressure can have a decided negative effect on therapy if the client feels that his peers disapprove of his receiving therapy. He feels that he is considered "different" or "handicapped" when he is taken out of the educational program to go for therapy. This goes against the peer pressure to fit in with the group and to be accepted by the group.

If the client is teased about his voice by his peers in the school environment, it can be extremely devastating, since this is the social environment in which he operates. Further, he is in competition with

—NOTES—

these peers academically and socially and his voice disorder interferes with this competition in both areas. His classroom performance will more than likely suffer because of his reluctance to speak in class. He is also handicapped as he attempts to compete socially. You should be aware of this potential negative influence on your therapy and, if problems do arise, you should be prepared to do some counseling.

Chapter 9

Vocal Behavioral Disorders

It was stressed in Chapter 3, Vocal Mechanics, that normal voice is the result of an interaction of several behaviors. Further, all the behaviors must be present and appropriately performed in order for normal voice to be produced. Each behavior, if deviant, can by itself produce a vocal disorder. Therefore, we will consider each behavior as a separate entity, keeping in mind however that many vocal disorders are the result of two or more improperly performed vocal behaviors. The following vocal behaviors are presented in their natural order of building voice.

BREATHING PATTERNS

Behaviors

The two deviant breathing patterns found in clients who have voice disorders are opposition breathing and clavicular breathing. In opposition breathing the thorax and the abdomen are out of phase in the respiratory cycle. In other words, as the thorax is in the inhalation phase and expanding, the abdomen is in an exhalation phase and compressing. The effect of opposition breathing is to reduce the lung's vital capacity and this is reflected in reduced breath support of the voice.

In order to compensate for the reduced vital capacity and breath support, people often resort to clavicular breathing. In this form of breathing, the rib cage is elevated by contraction of the strap muscles of the neck, pulling up the clavicle and the first rib. When the rib cage is thus "hyperelevated," the vital capacity is increased. Clavicular breathing is most often found accompanying opposition breathing. Since opposition breathing reduces the air supply, clavicular breathing is used to compensate by increasing the air supply.

—NOTES—

Vocal Problems

Although not a serious problem, incorrect breathing behaviors can contribute to vocal disorders. Because of increased tension in the neck, persons who use opposition and clavicular breathing and who do a considerable amount of loud speaking or yelling are susceptible to developing vocal nodes. Their incorrect respiratory habits and the resultant tension in the strap muscles are part of the total vocal abuse picture.

Others with incorrect breathing patterns may manifest a "weak" voice, that is, a voice that is too soft. These people just do not have an adequate air supply and subglottal air pressure to speak at a normal level. Teachers may report that a particular student talks so softly that no one can hear him and this may be directly related to a breathing problem. Many teenagers are sensitive about being "different" from their peers. If they are exceptionally tall, they may adjust their posture to camouflage it. The posture change, usually a slump of the shoulders forward, can inhibit normal breathing behaviors, and the result is insufficient breath support for speech. Posture is very important for proper breathing.

Overview

Auditory Orientation. Voice texts organized around auditory labels of vocal disorders would more than likely discuss the voice resulting from this behavioral disorder under the following headings:

> Weak voice
> Soft voice
> Disorders of vocal loudness

Medical Orientation. Voice texts organized around medical causes would more than likely discuss this vocal behavior disorder under the following headings:

> Respiration
> Asthma
> Emphysema

CHECKING ACTION

Behaviors

Checking action is defined as the prolonging of an exhalation by slowly relaxing the the muscles of inhalation as exhalation proceeds.

In this way the act of exhalation is controlled over a period of time, which is vital for appropriate speech. If checking action did not occur, the air from the lungs would rush out under great pressure at the onset of speech and the speaker would quickly run out of air. As a result, the speech at the beginning of the utterance would be louder than that at the end and the utterance would be very short.

Vocal Problems

When checking action is not appropriate, problems with voicing may be present. The most obvious problem is that of decreasing loudness during speech, with the speech becoming very soft at the end of utterances as the individual runs out of air. These utterances are also short in duration owing to lack of air. A problem of vocal quality may also be present, particularly at the onset of speech, when a rapid escape of air because of high subglottal air pressure occurs. The voice quality might also change toward the end of the utterance as the air supply is exhausted.

Overview

Auditory Orientation. Voice texts organized around auditory labels of vocal disorders would more than likely discuss the voice resulting from this behavioral disorder under the following headings:

Weak voice
Soft voice
Disorders of vocal loudness

Medical Orientation. Voice texts organized around medical causes would more than likely discuss this vocal behavior disorder under the following headings:

Neurological disorders
Respiration
Cerebral palsy
Hysterical/psychological disorders

VOCAL FOLD APPROXIMATION (INADEQUATE)

Behaviors

Either one or both of the vocal folds fail to approximate for normal voicing. If only one vocal fold fails to move properly, the other, when reaching its proper position, will not have the opposite vocal fold present to a complete the voicing approximation. The medial position of the vocal folds may vary from a very slight discrepancy in approximation to complete lack of approximation, in which both folds fail to move medially from their lateral position.

Vocal Problems

When the vocal folds fail to approximate correctly, air is allowed to pass between the vocal folds without being clearly modified into individual puffs of air. Thus, depending on the degree of movement, the listener can hear air escaping in addition to some basic vocal tone. The efficiency of the vocal fold vibrations is greatly reduced and is manifested in poor utilization of the air supply. In addition, because of inadequate approximation, there is a lack of subglottal air pressure, which results in problems with the loudness of the voice.

Overview

Auditory Orientation. Voice texts organized around auditory labels of vocal disorders would more than likely discuss the voice resulting from this behavioral disorder under the following headings:

Aphonia
Breathy voice
Weak voice
Soft voice
Hoarse voice
Whispered voice

Medical Orientation. Voice texts organized around medical causes would more than likely discuss this vocal behavior disorder under the following headings:

Vocal fold paralysis
Neurological disorders
Organic disorders
Hysterical/psychological disorders

VOCAL FOLD APPROXIMATION (EXCESSIVE)
Behaviors

In this instance the vocal folds, instead of only approximating, pass the point of approximation and close tightly into the breath-holding position. This action must involve both vocal folds, and their degree of closure would range from slight to extreme.

Vocal Problems

When the vocal folds are closed into the breath-holding position, the subglottal air pressure must build quite high to override the tension in the vocal folds in order to make them vibrate. When this occurs, the vocal tone is quite loud, and because the vocal folds spend more time in the closed phase than in the open phase, the vocal quality reflects the high level of tension used in vocal production. The restricted vibratory action of the vocal folds also interferes with normal use of the air supply. In some instances the subglottal air pressure is only partially successful in overriding the laryngeal tension and vibrating the vocal folds. In this situation the individual's voice consists mainly of "squeaks," sometimes separated by periods of silence.

Overview

Auditory Orientation. Voice texts organized around auditory labels of vocal disorders would more than likely discuss the voice resulting from this behavioral disorder under the following headings:

Harsh voice
Grating voice
Strident voice
Strangled voice
Spastic voice
Raspy voice

Medical Orientation. Voice texts organized around medical causes would more than likely discuss this vocal behavior disorder under the following headings:

Spastic dysphonia
Hysterical/psychological disorders

VOCAL FOLD VIBRATION (ASYNCHRONOUS)

Behaviors

In normal vibration, each vocal fold vibrates at the same frequency, thus creating an efficient vibrating system. If for some reason one vocal fold has a different muscular tonus, mass, or length, that vocal fold will vibrate at a frequency different from the other fold. This irregularity in vocal fold vibration disrupts the normally efficient system.

Vocal Problems

When a lack of regular, synchronous vibration of the vocal folds is present, air is allowed to escape without being modified into "puffs," and this is heard as a high pitched noise, giving the voice a "breathy" component. In addition, since the folds are vibrating at different frequencies, this results in a low pitched noise, adding an irregular or "rough" component to the voice. In many instances both high and low pitched noise is heard in the vocal quality.

Overview

Auditory Orientation. Voice texts organized around auditory labels of vocal disorders would more than likely discuss the voice resulting from this behavioral disorder under the following headings:

Hoarse voice
Rough voice

Medical Orientation. Voice texts organized around medical causes would more than likely discuss this vocal behavior disorder under the following headings:

Vocal nodes
Vocal ulcers
Polyps
Laryngitis
Neurological disorders
Vocal fold paralysis

VOCAL FOLD VIBRATION (VARIABLE)

Behaviors

Under these conditions, the vocal folds vary in their mode of vibration, from inadequate to excessive closure, from synchronous to asynchronous movements, or a combination of both. These changes in the vibratory mode of the vocal folds occur randomly during vocalization.

Vocal Problems

As the vocal folds change their mode of vibration, the efficiency of the vibration shifts from allowing too much air to escape, to preventing air from escaping, to asynchronous vibrations, to synchronous vibrations. The voice varies accordingly, shifting from one form of inefficient system to another but never stabilizing. The listener hears vocal disorders associated with inadequate or excessive vocal fold approximation and with synchronous or asynchronous vocal fold vibrations.

Overview

Auditory Orientation. Voice texts organized around auditory labels of vocal disorders would more than likely discuss the voice resulting from this behavioral disorder under the following headings:

Spastic voice

Medical Orientation. Voice texts organized around medical causes would more than likely discuss this vocal behavior disorder under the following headings:

Spastic dysphonia
Hysterical/psychological disorders
Cerebral palsy
Neurological disorders

LARYNGEAL LENGTH/TENSION/MASS (L/T/M) ADJUSTMENTS

Behaviors

Muscular adjustments in the larynx vary the length, the tension, and the mass of the vocal folds. These adjustments determine the frequency of vibration of the vocal folds. When the folds are elongated, their mass is decreased as their tension is increased. This results in a raising of the pitch. As the folds are shortened, their mass increases as their tension is decreased and the pitch is lowered.

Vocal Problems

If the L/T/M adjustments are not appropriate, the pitch level of the voice may be too high or too low for the individual. Furthermore, if these adjustments are restricted, the individual may have a narrow pitch range, that is, a monopitch voice. If on the other hand the adjustments are too extensive and inappropriate, the pitch range might be too variable.

Overview

Auditory Orientation. Voice texts organized around auditory labels of vocal disorders would more than likely discuss the voice resulting from this behavioral disorder under the following headings:

Disorders of vocal pitch

Medical Orientation. Voice texts organized around medical causes would more than likely discuss this vocal behavior disorder under the following headings:

Normal development
Psychological/hysterical disorders
Neurological disorders
Cerebral palsy

LARYNGEAL COMPRESSION ADJUSTMENTS

Behaviors

Muscular adjustments in the larynx "compress" the larynx around the vocal folds, increasing their resistance to vibration. This resistance increases the amount of subglottal air pressure needed to make the folds vibrate. As subglottal air pressure increases, so does the loudness of the voice. In some instances, even though the vocal folds are approximated for vocalization, because of muscular weakness they are "bowed" and allow air to escape.

Vocal Problems

If the compression adjustments are inappropriate, the loudness level of the voice may be too soft or too loud. Furthermore, if these adjustments are restricted, the individual may have a narrow loudness range, that is, a "monoloudness" voice. If on the other hand the adjustments are too extensive and inappropriate, the loudness range might be too variable.

Overview

Auditory Orientation. Voice texts organized around auditory labels of vocal disorders would more than likely discuss the voice resulting from this behavioral disorder under the following headings:

Weak voice
Soft voice
Breathy voice
Harsh voice
Strident voice

Medical Orientation. Voice texts organized around medical causes would more than likely discuss this vocal behavior disorder under the following headings:

Normal development
Psychological/hysterical disorders
Neurological disorders
Gerontology
Cerebral palsy
Auditory disorders

LARYNGEAL ADJUSTMENT COORDINATION

Behaviors

The adjustments in the larynx for pitch and for loudness are independent behaviors. The pitch of the voice can be altered without changing the loudness and vice versa. However, the interaction between pitch and loudness is an integral part of vocal prosody. Thus, if the pitch and loudness adjustments are not independent, or are inadequate for some other reason, the normal prosody of the voice is disturbed.

Vocal Problems

If the laryngeal adjustments are not coordinated, the individual may have inappropriate prosody, which would interfere with the contextual aspects of communication. The problem now takes on aspects of a language disorder.

Overview

Auditory Orientation. Voice texts organized around auditory labels of vocal disorders would more than likely discuss the voice resulting from this behavioral disorder under the following headings:

Disorders of prosody
Dialect/accent

Medical Orientation. Voice texts organized around medical causes would more than likely discuss this vocal behavior disorder under the following headings:

Psychological/hysterical disorders
Neurological disorders
Cerebral palsy
Auditory disorders

RESONANCE COUPLING

Behaviors

Resonance of the voice is a complex issue. We will limit our discussion to the role of nasal resonance in voice quality. Nasal resonance results from the opening of the nasopharyngeal port, accomplished basically by the lowering of the soft palate. When the port is closed by the raising of the soft palate, the nasal resonator is sealed off from the vocal tract.

Vocal Problems

If the nasopharyngeal port remains open or does not achieve a proper seal during speech, excessive nasal resonance is present in the voice. Also, if the timing of the opening and closing of the port is sluggish or poorly coordinated, there will be some spread of nasal resonance to sounds preceding and following the nasalized sound. Both of these deviations are usually referred to as hypernasality.

If on the other hand the port between the nasal cavity and the oral cavity is blocked so that sound can not enter the nasal cavity, there will be a lack of appropriate nasal resonance, or hyponasality. In some instances, hyponasality is viewed as an articulation disorder, since only the nasal sounds are involved.

Overview

Auditory Orientation. Voice texts organized around auditory labels of vocal disorders would more than likely discuss the voice resulting from this behavioral disorder under the following headings:

Nasality
Hypernasality
Hyponasality
Articulation disorders

Medical Orientation. Voice texts organized around medical causes would more than likely discuss this vocal behavior disorder under the following headings:

Normal development
Neurological disorders
Cleft palate
Deviated septum
Polyps
Adenoids

Chapter 10

Getting the New Behavior to Occur

ANTECEDENT AND CONTINGENT EVENTS

We are now ready to begin teaching the client to produce a new vocal behavior. In our interactions with the client we will be using the CIM model. This means we will be paying particular attention to antecedent and contingent events as we teach. We will carefully present antecedent events in the form of modeling, information, and guidance so that the client knows what we want him to learn. He knows the behavior change goal. When he performs in a way that indicates that he is learning to perform the new behavior, we will reward him. This contingent event is vital to our teaching and learning interactions with the client. Because the client is just learning to perform the new behavior, we will reward every occurrence of the new behavior. This continuous reward schedule encourages rapid learning. Each clinical transaction will be a test of how well the client is learning. We will gradually shape the new behavior to the appropriate form for normal vocal production or to the limits imposed by any possible intervening factor such as a medical or structural problem.

CLINICAL TECHNIQUES (a.k.a. STRATEGIES)

What does every clinician wish for? A recipe book—a book filled with every conceivable recipe for teaching every conceivable thing to every conceivable type of client. Recipes are in; creativity and inventiveness are out. This appears to apply to cooking as well as it does to voice therapy. Everyone who cooks either wants or has a recipe for everything. Take stew for example. What is the mystery about stew? There are only three ingredients: meat, vegetables, and spices. You put them together in some combination and, after they cook, you have stew. It really is that simple. But there must be at least 10,000 recipes for stew, and 5000 of them are for Irish stew. Now, really, what is a recipe

—NOTES—

for stew? It is no more than a combination of ingredients that someone else tried and thought tasted good so they wrote down how much of what they put together.

Clinical techniques are just recipes for "clinical stew." There are three ingredients: modeling, information, and guidance, and all the techniques that people write about are just their teaching recipes that they think work reasonably well. They took a dash of modeling, a pinch of information, and a cup of guidance, and after mixing and letting it cook in the client's head for a while, they found that the client learned. So, they wrote down the recipe so others could use their "clinical stew." But who is to say that the other therapist-cooks have the best recipes? You have all the ingredients; make your own recipe. You have some choices, just as you do when you make Irish stew (what kind of meat, vegetables, and spices you are going to use). As a therapist, you must decide what kind of modeling you are going to use and how much you will put in. And what are the kinds of information you are going to put in? Guidance, your spice, has several forms for you to chose from. Put your clinical stew together and taste test it on your clients. You are not going to poison anyone. Who knows, you may discover the most outstanding stew in the world for your therapy. Then you can publish your recipe for the rest of the world's recipe collectors. We will give you a few recipes as we discuss teaching the new vocal behaviors, but it is up to you to expand your clinical techniques. As you develop your techniques you will find they can be applied to all clients, not just the voice client.

BREATHING PATTERNS

Clinical Goal. To re-establish the normal breathing pattern.

Clinical Rationale. Opposition breathing cannot occur if the correct breathing pattern is used since the two forms of breathing are mutually exclusive. Therefore, by concentrating on teaching correct breathing behaviors, the incorrect pattern will automatically be eliminated. Once the correct breathing pattern has replaced the opposition breathing, clavicular breathing will no longer occur because it is no longer needed.

Teaching Strategies:

Modeling. Have the client observe you as you demonstrate the correct movements of the thorax and abdomen during respiration.

Information. Explain to the client that the thorax and abdomen should move together in respiration, that is, they both move outward during inhalation and inward during exhalation.

Guidance
1. Place your hand on the client's stomach during his attempts to breathe properly and press the stomach in during exhalation. Do this while the client is standing.
2. Have the client lie down, place his hand on his stomach, and practice the correct breathing. After the client can do this while lying down, have him stand and repeat it.

CHECKING ACTION

Clinical Goal. To improve the client's checking action so he can maintain his air flow over time.

Clinical Rationale. Checking action is a natural part of respiration and is always present. The checking action required for speech is only an extension of normal checking action. Therefore, there is no need to teach a new behavior, only to extend the ability of an existing behavior. If the checking action is absent, the client has more serious problems than a voice disorder.

Teaching Strategies:

Modeling. Have the client observe you as you extend an exhalation.

Information. Tell the client to bring his chest down and his stomach in slowly as he exhales and to let as little air out as possible and still be exhaling.

Guidance
1. Have the client hold his hand in front of your mouth as you extend an exhalation so he can feel how long your exhalation is. Then have him hold his hand in front of his own mouth as he attempts to extend the duration of his own exhalation.
2. Use a stop watch to let the client know how long his exhalations are and how successful he is in extending their duration.
3. Hold a mirror in front of the client's mouth and see how long he can maintain the steam on the mirror.

VOCAL FOLD APPROXIMATION
(INADEQUATE/ORGANIC)

Clinical Goal. To improve the client's ability to approximate the vocal folds.

Clinical Rationale. Because this client has an organic (medical) problem that is preventing him from approximating the vocal folds, there is little that can be done to improve the behavioral performance. If the medical problem is reversible, therapy should not be planned until the client has completed the medical program and the voice can be evaluated under these new conditions. If the medical problem is not reversible, only limited clinical gains can be expected. In order to compensate for the lack of approximation, laryngeal tension must be increased if possible.

Teaching Strategies:

Modeling. Demonstrate laryngeal tension by tensing the strap muscles in your neck. You can do this by pushing your head back with your hand and resisting the movement by tensing the neck muscles.

Information. Explain to the client what you are trying to accomplish. You might even show him anatomical drawings of the larynx, including illustrations of how the vocal folds close.

Guidance
1. Have the client feel his neck as he attempts to tense his muscles.
2. Compress the larynx gently with your fingers as the client attempts to produce a vocal tone.
3. Have the client tilt his head as far forward or backward as he can while attempting to produce a vocal tone.
4. Have the client attempt to lift the seat of his chair while he is seated on it. Encourage him to grunt while attempting this.

VOCAL FOLD APPROXIMATION
(INADEQUATE/FUNCTIONAL)

Clinical Goal. To improve the client's ability to approximate the vocal folds.

Clinical Rationale. Because there is no organic or physical reason why the vocal folds are not approximated, we can assume that the inability to perform this behavior is emotional in nature. If very obvious emotional problems seem to be involved in the behavioral problem and the resultant voice quality, a referral for counseling is in order. However, if the client has assumed this behavior because of social rewards associated with the resultant voice quality (such as a sexy, breathy voice), but in your opinion this vocal behavior might lead to more serious vocal problems, this client should receive therapy. The main focus in therapy will be to introduce tension into the larynx, but some general counseling should also be given.

There is a fine line between those clients who are referred for counseling and those who can benefit from direct voice therapy. It is important that you recognize that you have the ability to do limited counseling with your clients. It is for this reason that the chapter on counseling was included in this book.

Teaching Strategies:

Modeling. Demonstrate laryngeal tension by tensing the strap muscles in your neck. You can do this by pushing your head back with your hand and resisting the movement by tensing the neck muscles.

Information. Explain to the client what you are trying to accomplish. You might even show him anatomical drawings of the larynx, including illustrations of how the vocal folds close. He needs to understand the role of muscular contraction and muscular tension as related to approximating the folds.

Guidance
1. Have the client feel his neck as he attempts to tense his muscles.
2. Compress the larynx gently with your fingers as the client attempts to produce a vocal tone.
3. Have the client tilt his head as far forward or backward as he can while attempting to produce a vocal tone.
4. Have the client attempt to lift the seat of his chair while he is sitting on it. Encourage him to grunt while attempting this.

VOCAL FOLD APPROXIMATION (EXCESSIVE)

Clinical Goal. To have the client approximate the vocal folds without undue tension.

Clinical Rationale. We know of no organic reason for prolonged excessive approximation of the vocal folds for voicing. We must assume therefore that it is a learned, emotional response, perhaps a laryn-

—NOTES—

geal reflection of general body tension. In some instances this kind of client might better be served through counseling than with direct voice therapy. However, for the most part, these clients can be treated by providing them with a means of relaxing the strap muscles and teaching them to perform an easy vocal onset.

Teaching Strategies:

Modeling. Model both behaviors you are teaching. Contrast easy with hard vocal onset. Model neck relaxation by rolling the head or hanging it down on your chest.

Information. Explain carefully to the client how tension in the neck and larynx affects vocal production. Make certain he understands how tension in strap muscles can influence the tension levels of the muscles in the larynx and inhibit their movements. Explain very carefully how the vocal folds approximate for voice but do not close. The client should understand the difference between vocalizing and holding the breath.

Guidance
1. Have the client produce the [h] sound and gradually introduce a vowel, for example, as in the work *hay.*
2. Have the client produce a prolonged vowel sound and vary the vocal pitch and loudness during the vowel production so that the muscular movement will bring about some relaxation.
3. Have the client attempt to produce a "breathy" voice, a vocal production in which you can hear air escaping between the vocal folds.
4. Guide the client through the steps of one of the methods of relaxation presented in Appendix B.

VOCAL FOLD VIBRATION (ASYNCHRONOUS)

Clinical Goal. To make the vocal folds vibrate in a regular, synchronous manner.

Clinical Rationale. There are two main reasons for irregular vocal fold vibration: paralysis and mass imbalances. Paralysis is better dealt with in the section Vocal Fold Approximation (Inadequate/Organic). We will deal here with problems due to mass imbalances. Variations in mass, either as growths or edema, are usually attributable to some form of vocal abuse. In order to achieve regular vibrations of the vocal folds, the added mass must be eliminated. Therefore, the clinical approach to this disorder will be to eliminate vocal behaviors that abuse the vocal folds. If improper breathing patterns are a factor, they should be dealt with according to the procedures put forth in the section Breathing Patterns.

Teaching Strategies:

Modeling. Depending on the vocal behaviors the client is using, you may be modeling (1) appropriate opening and closing of the vocal folds, (2) appropriate pitch level, (3) appropriate pitch and loudness interaction, or (4) any combination of these.

Information. Vocal abuse is the result of a complex series of behaviors and events, and the client must understand how together they are irritating the vocal folds to the point at which they are changing physiologically. He must understand that by removing the vocal abuse, the vocal folds will return to their normal state and, more than likely, the vocal disorder will correct itself. He may also need to be informed about the surgical approach to the removal of vocal nodes. This information may be important to his motivation.

Guidance. Guide the client through the appropriate steps of the program for Vocal Hygiene found in Appendix C.

VOCAL FOLD VIBRATION (VARIABLE)

Clinical Goal. To enable the client to produce a steady vocal tone while maintaining quality, pitch, and loudness.

Clinical Rationale. Because laryngeal approximation or vibrational mode is variable in this type of client, we will probably be dealing either with an organic factor such as that found in a cerebral palsied child or with a psychogenic disorder such as spastic dysphonia. In either event, we are faced with "spasms" in the larynx that create the variable mode of vibration. Our best approach to this problem would be to work on relaxation to reduce the extent and effect of the spasms, since there appears to be no way to eliminate the spasms themselves.

Teaching strategies:

Modeling. Demonstrate neck relaxation by rolling the head or hanging it down on your chest.

—NOTES—

Information. Explain to the client how muscles, when held in a state of contraction over a period of time, go into spasms and how, by relaxing them, the spasms can be reduced. Go into enough detail about the relaxation method so that the client understands the process.

Guidance. Guide the client through the steps of one of the methods of relaxation found in Appendix B.

LARYNGEAL LENGTH/TENSION/MASS (L/T/M) ADJUSTMENTS

Clinical Goal. To establish an appropriate pitch level for the client.

Clinical Rationale. Pitch level is a subjective judgment. Levels may vary considerably among people and not create problems. However, when the male pitch level is judged too high or the female pitch judged too low by listeners, certain undesirable social implications result. When this occurs, the individual with the variant pitch level has a vocal problem. A more appropriate pitch level must be established for the individual.

The pitch range can also be a problem, particularly if the pitch varies in extremes. This type of pitch problem is best dealt with under the previous section, Vocal Fold Vibration (Variable).

Teaching Strategies

Modeling. Demonstrate the appropriate pitch level for the client. You may need a pitch pipe in order to be able to reproduce the pitch. You should also contrast the appropriate pitch with the pitch the client is using.

Information. You should explain that the vocal folds have a natural pitch based on their size and that the pitch the client uses is not the natural pitch for his vocal folds. He needs to understand that the purpose of therapy is to establish a pitch level that is closer to the natural pitch of his vocal folds.

Guidance

1. Establish the natural pitch by having the client "sing" the lowest note he can and then have him go up the scale four notes (do, re, me, fa). This should be close to the natural pitch. In some instances you will feel the pitch is more natural if you go up five notes instead of four.

2. Hum the proper pitch or play the appropriate note on a pitch pipe

softly as the client attempts to say short phrases at the indicated pitch.
3. As the client speaks, provide him with gestural feedback about the appropriateness of his pitch. Pointing the finger up means to raise the pitch, whereas pointing the finger down means to lower the pitch.

LARYNGEAL COMPRESSION ADJUSTMENTS

Clinical Goal. To establish an appropriate vocal loudness level for the client.

Clinical Rationale. In many instances, disorders of loudness are handled with procedures dealing with vocal fold approximation, since a behavior disorder of loudness rarely occurs in isolation except with auditory impairment, emotional involvement, general muscular weakness, or because of reward for this type of vocal behavior. With an auditory disorder the client's vocal problems are much more pervasive than just loudness and are not considered here. If the loud voice is a manifestation of a deep emotional problem, we must make an appropriate referral. The extremely weak voice associated with muscular weakness is only part of a much more involved problem. However, if the behavior exists because it has been rewarded, perhaps as part of a personality, we can work with the motivated client to modify this behavior. Our therapy might include some counseling.

Teaching Strategies:

Modeling. You should model both inappropriate and appropriate loudness of speech for the client so he can distinguish between them. This may be either too loud or too soft a voice.

Information. The client should understand the role of muscular tension in the production of voice. It should also be made clear how too little or too much tension affects vocal production and the vocal folds themselves. When appropriate the concept of vocal abuse and misuse should be introduced (Appendix C).

Guidance
1. Set the recording meter (the volume unit [VU] meter) on your tape recorder so it registers 0 at what you would consider a normal loudness level. Have the client speak into the microphone from the same distance you did and have him keep the meter at "0." When he can do this, keep moving him further back

from the microphone and have him adjust his loudness accordingly.

2. If the client is speaking at an inappropriate loudness level, give him a gesture that he understands to mean adjust the loudness accordingly; for example, pointing up means to make the speech louder and pointing down means to speak more softly.

LARYNGEAL ADJUSTMENT COORDINATION

Clinical Goal. To create appropriate vocal prosody that reflects the linguistic content intended by the client.

Clinical Rationale. If the prosody of the voice does not truly reflect the intended contextual content of the linguistic unit of the client, the vocal problem is manifesting itself both as a vocal and a language disorder. A disorder of prosody disrupts the relationship between content and context of linguistic messages in normal communication. In order to re-establish prosody, the client must learn to coordinate the independent laryngeal functions of changing the pitch and the loudness of the voice.

Teaching Strategies:

Modeling. Model various prosodic forms of a sentence as the client identifies the linguistic form. You should also model the independence of pitch and loudness (changing pitch while maintaining loudness and vice versa).

Information. Explain what "prosody" means: how pitch and loudness interact to stress words and give melody to speech for meaning. Explain various linguistic forms dependent on prosody.

Guidance
1. After planning a phrase, change the linguistic meaning by guiding the client through hand gestures to change the prosody as the phrase is repeated.
2. Write out a series of questions and change the prosody by underlining different words in each question.
3. Have the client make a series of statements and guide the stress he gives to certain words through hand gestures.

RESONANCE COUPLING

Clinical Goal. To establish an appropriate amount of nasal resonance in the client's voice.

Clinical Rationale. Because we are approaching this clinical situation as a voice problem, we will exclude cleft palate, viewing this as a separate clinical entity. We are then dealing with the client who cannot completely seal off the nasal resonator or the child whose timing of closure is not appropriate, so there is spread of nasal resonance to surrounding sounds. We must either improve the client's ability to close the nasopharyngeal port or increase the speed of his closure. Our clinical task is to strengthen the muscles involved in this action and improve their coordination.

Teaching Strategies:

Modeling. Read a series of sentences demonstrating both normal and excessive nasality. Produce a variety of syllables normally and then with excessive nasality.

Information. Explain to the client that there are only three phonemes in our language that must have nasal resonance and that all of the other sounds can be produced normally with no nasal resonance. Also explain the timing necessary to introduce the nasal resonance only when the nasalized sound is being produced and the removal of the resonance as soon as the nasalized sound is completed.

Guidance
1. Have the client repeat the syllable [mpɑ] while attempting to achieve palatal closure and then make the repetition faster as closure occurs.
2. Have the client suck water through a straw. Extend the length of the straw as the client succeeds.
3. Have the client imitate snoring.

STIMULUS MANIPULATION

Role Shift. Because this is the first phase of therapy and you are just entering a clinical relationship with your client, you come into therapy with no stimulus value: You are an S0. You will assume an S+

role as soon as the client associates you with the rewards he is receiving from you in therapy. Once you assume this role you will prompt or cue the new vocal behavior when the client is with you. When it comes time for you to correct his production and give him some negative feedback (a penalty), you will assume the S− role, cuing or prompting the client not to perform the incorrect behavior so as to avoid the penalty. These clinical stimulus roles will continue during this phase of therapy.

Gradual Introduction of Stimuli. If you can simply provide the model of the new behavior (your stimulus) and the client is able to produce it, this is the most efficient form of therapy. However, if this does not succeed, gradually add more to your stimulus. Make the model more complete or longer in duration. If this also fails, add information and then finally add guidance. Make the stimulus only as complex as necessary for the client. Do not overwhelm the client with a complex stimulus when all he might need is a simple model.

Gradual Withdrawal of Stimuli. As the client begins to produce the desired behavior, you should begin to withdraw your stimulus. Do this gradually by making the stimulus less complex. Your goal in this phase of therapy is to have the behavior occur without a model or guidance.

Increasing the Number of Stimuli. We are using this form of stimulus manipulation very simply in this phase of therapy. We are increasing the number of stimuli as we make our clinical stimulus more complex. We are also increasing the number of S+ by assuming this role as a result of rewarding the new behavior.

Decreasing the Number of Stimuli. The only way that this form of manipulation is involved is our gradual withdrawal of the clinical stimulus.

Chapter 11

Stabilizing and Generalizing the New Behavior

STABILIZING THE NEW VOCAL BEHAVIOR

Antecedent and Contingent Events

We gradually eliminated the antecedent events of modeling, information, and guidance during the last phase of therapy and shifted our attention to the contingent events of rewards, rewarding every occurrence of the new vocal behavior. As we move into this phase of therapy our clinical focus shifts from the continuous presentation of reward for behavioral performance to the gradual withdrawal of the reward. The gradual withdrawal of the reward is your clinical test of the stability of the behavior. As the behavior becomes more stabilized, that is, more natural and spontaneous for the client, it is less dependent on the external reward. The withdrawal of the contingent reward should be gradual. When we move from rewarding every occurrence of the behavior to every other performance, we have reduced the reward system by 50 percent. This is a major change in the reward schedule. It might be better to move from rewarding every performance to 9 out of 10 performances. This is a 10 percent reduction and should not have any major impact on the client. Continue this gradual removal of rewards until the behavior is stabilized and naturally occurring in the client's vocal productions.

In the event that the behavioral performance slips a bit, back up in therapy until the behavior is stable again. This may mean that you have to present some antecedent events such as modeling or guidance and you may even have to go back to a continuous reward schedule. This will create no clinical problems. However, as soon as the behavior is stable again, withdraw the antecedent events and start withdrawing reward again. Remember that human learning is not a steady, constantly progressing process. It has its ups and downs. This is why human learning is referred to as "saw-toothed" in nature. However, the direction of the learning must, in the long run, be a progressive process.

Stimulus Manipulation

Role Shift. You are now serving as an S+ to cue the new behavior in the client and an S− to cue the client not to perform the deviant behavior. As you progressed through the first phase of therapy the instances in which the client could not perform the new behavior became fewer and fewer, indicating that the client was indeed learning. As a result, your S− role faded, since there were very few instances for which you had to provide the client with negative feedback (penalty). Your S+ remained very strong because you continued to provide continuous rewards.

As you proceed through this phase of therapy your S+ role will fade and you provide fewer and fewer rewards. In other words, if you only reward 50 percent of the behavioral performances, you are assuming the S0 role for the remaining 50 percent of the performances. By the end of this phase of therapy you should shift your clinical role to that of an S0, not cuing or prompting the new behavior for a reward. The behavior will still occur regularly, since it is stable and the client habitually uses the behavior when talking to you.

Gradual Introduction of Stimuli. Gradual introduction of stimuli is not used in this phase of therapy.

Gradual Withdrawal of Stimuli. Gradual withdrawl of stimuli is not used in this phase of therapy except as you gradually withdraw the reward.

Decreasing the Number of Stimuli. As you shift your roles from S+ and S− to an S0 you are decreasing the number of positive and negative stimuli.

Increasing the Number of Stimuli. Increasing the number of stimuli is not used in this phase of therapy.

Integrating New Vocal Behaviors into Speech

As the new behavior becomes more stable in this phase of therapy, the behavior should be integrated into speech production within the clinical environment. For example, if vocal fold approximation has been improved in the prolonging of a vowel sound, the new behavior should now be attempted as the client produces speech segments of increasing duration. Another example would be a client whose habitual pitch level, the pitch level he spoke at before therapy, was lowered to a more appropriate level. At first the client will only be able to utter short phrases while maintaining the new pitch level. During this phase of therapy the new pitch level should be stabilized in the client's speech in the clinical environment.

GENERALIZING THE NEW VOCAL BEHAVIOR

Antecedent and Contingent Events

In the last step in therapy we focused our attention on the contingent events, primarily on the rewards administered to clients. At this point in therapy, the new vocal behavior is occurring consistently in the clinical environment. The problem now is that the behavior has not been generalized to other talking environments. In other words, the behavior is being used only in the clinical environment: When the client is with the clinician, the behavior is habituated, but when the clinician is not present, nothing cues the new behavior to occur. The clinician must now concentrate on generalizing the new vocal behavior to all speaking environments.

Since the clinical goal in this phase of therapy is to make the new behavior occur in other speaking environments, we shift our clinical focus to the antecedent events, the stimuli that prompt or cue the behavior to occur. We will manipulate these stimuli in such ways as to increase the S+ that prompts the behavior. Of course, at the same time we will provide rewards for the client as he performs the new behavior in these new environments. One way to view this phase of therapy is that, in essence, we are repeating the first phase of therapy, getting the new behavior to occur, but this time we are concentrating on getting the behavior to occur in other speech environments.

Stimulus Manipulation

Role Shift. You are now an S0 for the new behavior. It is stable in the clinical environment without your rewards. Your S− role has disappeared, since there are no longer occurrences of the incorrect behavior for you to penalize. You will continue this role as associated with the new behavior, but you will now take on a new S+ role through your rewarding the client for his performing the new behavior outside the therapy environment. Also, if you have a means of checking on

—NOTES—

his performance outside, you may assume an S— role for failure to use the new behavior in other speaking situations.

It is now time to bring significant others into the clinical picture. One of our clinical goals in this phase of therapy is to increase the number of S+ in the client's speaking environments to prompt the new vocal behavior. Significant others can assume the role of S+ by providing rewards for the new behavior. Once the association is made between them and the rewards, they become an S+ and prompt the behavior to occur.

We also want to increase the number of S+ talking situations, situations that cue or prompt the new vocal behavior to occur. One of the ways we accomplish this is to shift S— talking situations to S+ situations. As we shift the roles of situations, we are also increasing the number of S+ and decreasing the number of S—.

Gradual Introduction of Stimuli. With certain kinds of clients there might well be speaking situations that are so frightening that they are an S—, preventing the occurrence of the new behavior by creating extreme tension in the client. We may have to present these situations gradually to give the client an opportunity to adjust to them. An example would be an adolescent male with a new lower vocal pitch. He may find it extremely embarrassing to speak to a class of peers with the new pitch. We might begin the introduction of the new pitch by having him use it with one male peer in the therapy environment. Once it is occurring with one listener, another male listener can be added. The third listener could be a female peer. As we gradually introduce the client to speaking to a group of peers, the fear associated with speaking to a class of peers is reduced. As we reduce the fear, we are increasing the probability that he will be able to perform the new pitch.

Gradual Withdrawal of Stimuli. There are only very special instances in which this strategy would be used in this stage of therapy. Also, we are referring to a highly specialized type of stimulus we would be withdrawing. This situation can best be presented in the form of an illustration. Let us consider the same client we discussed in the last example, the male student with the new low pitch. The other clients in his shaping group have assumed an S+ role, since they have been rewarding his use of the new pitch in the group discussions. One of the frightening situations in which he finds he cannot use the new pitch is during recess in the gymnasium. He becomes so tense in this situation he cannot produce the new pitch, so this talking situation is an S—. One way we can better the client's chances of getting his new pitch to occur in the S— situation is to counter the negative influence of the

S − with the positive influence of an S +. In order to do this we would arrange for a group member to be with the client when he attempts to use his new pitch in the gymnasium. The group member, being an S +, should counteract the S − role of the talking situation and improve the client's ability to use the new pitch. After the new pitch has been introduced, the group member is gradually faded (withdrawn) from the situation. When the new pitch is used the second time, the group member is not standing as close to the client. With the third use the group member is standing quite far away. As the gymnasium situation shifts from an S − to an S +, the need for the S + support of the group member diminishes and it is withdrawn.

Decreasing the Number of Stimuli. If this form of stimulus manipulation is used, it must only be used to decrease the number of S − speaking situations a client might have. These frightening situations can be shifted from an S − role to either an S0 or an S + by changing the contingent event from penalty to reward. It might be necessary to present these situations gradually in order to achieve this role shift.

Increasing the Number of Stimuli. As you shift the roles of significant others, you are increasing the number of S +. This is vital to generalizing the new behavior to other environments (carry-over). As was stated earlier, one of the main problems we have as clinicians is to get the client to use his new communication behavior outside the clinical environment. Once the client is out of this environment and we are no longer present, the client just does not seem to be able to remember to use the new behavior. The old adage, "Out of sight, out of mind," applies here. Since we are not in the client's other speaking environments acting as an S + to cue or prompt the new behavior, we must attempt to find another S + to serve this purpose.

We know that we can create the S + role by associating the individual or the object with rewards. By associating the parents with rewards, we can shift them to an S + role to cue the behavior in the home environment. What about the school? If a teacher has the time to become associated with rewarding the client's behavior, even on an intermittent basis, she will become an S + for the classroom. Perhaps the most important resource we have is the shaping group. Each member of the group has been involved in rewarding all other group members so they are all an S +. This means that whenever they see each other in the school, the new behaviors are prompted to occur.

The more we plan our generalization of the new behavior and manipulate the client's environment, the more effective and efficient this phase of therapy will become. We would all agree that this phase of therapy is the most difficult and challenging for the speech clinician.

Specific Generalization Techniques

Reminders. Even with additional S+ in the client's environments, the main problem in generalizing the new behavior appears to be reminding the client to perform the behavior. The S+ are not always present and the client "forgets" to perform the new behavior, going back to performing the incorrect behavior because it is more habitual. A reminder is an object or event that is placed in the client's environment that calls his attention to his vocal behavior. For example, if a client whose voice was hypernasal wore his watch on the wrong wrist for a day, looking to see what time it was could serve to remind him to use the correct nasopharyngeal closure. Reminders are like tying a string around your finger to remember to do something. You can make up your own reminders but keep in mind that whatever is used must be rather obvious and something the client will be aware of during the day. Leaving a note on the dresser at home will not work except when the client wonders why the note is on the dresser.

Logbook. The logbook is no more than a small notebook the client carries with him to record the use of his new vocal behavior. In order to generalize the behavior in other speaking environments, the client must perform the behavior there. Therefore, he is given assignments to speak with the new behavior in specific environments. When he uses the behavior, he is to make a written record of his success so you can see it. Let us take an example.

This client, a 15 year old female, had a very breathy voice quality; that is, she did not completely approximate her vocal folds and you could hear air escaping. She did this because she felt it was attractive to the boys in her class and she wanted the attention. Her vocal behavior (lack of approximation) became habituated over time. She was referred to therapy because her voice was so soft she could not be heard by the teachers. A medical examination revealed that she was beginning to develop nodes because of the vocal abuse associated with the "whispered" speech. Appropriate approximation of the vocal folds was achieved in the clinical environment, but the client did not use the new behavior in social speaking situations. She was assigned to speak in two short speaking situations each day and to record her experiences in her logbook. She was to enter the following information in the logbook:

1. Enough information about the situation so that she could remember it to discuss it during her therapy session.
2. Assignment of a grade, *A* through *E*, that would reflect her success (or failure) to produce the new behavior and new voice quality.

3. Some sort of indication of how she felt about her new voice in the situation.
4. An assessment of how she felt her listener reacted to her new voice.

The information that is kept in the logbook varies according to the individual clinician, the individual client, the type of vocal disorder present, and so forth. The information in the logbook is there to be used by the clinician to reward the use of the new behavior; to make the client cognitively aware that the resultant vocal production is an asset and not a liability; to remind the client to use the new behavior; and to keep a record of the successful use of the new behavior in speaking situations outside the clinical environment.

The logbook would be of special value when working with a client whose problem is centered around vocal abuse. Here the situations would focus on the proper use of the voice in situations in which the client would normally abuse it. The client would pay special attention to proper use of the voice in recess, the gym, and other such environments. This might be of particular value for clients who are involved in cheerleading and are learning proper vocal behaviors in this situation.

Token Economy at Home. The use of a token economy at home is naturally dependent on parental cooperation, the seriousness of the vocal disorder, and the amount of time the clinician has to devote to the individual client. If these factors are all favorable, the token economy can be a most powerful tool for carry-over. With the parents providing the rewards through tokens, they assume very powerful S + roles outside the clinical environment. If the token economy you have set up also includes the removal of tokens for incorrect behavioral production, the parents also assume the S − role for the incorrect behavior. Perhaps of even greater importance is the motivation provided for the client. He will use his new vocal behavior in order to get more tokens to purchase the back-up reward. He will also avoid using the incorrect behavior if there is a penalty associated with its occurrence. The parents must remember to keep their "store" well stocked, since the first things the child will purchase are the most desirable for him. Therefore, as the store is emptied, the strength of the rewards diminishes.

Epilogue

The Referral and Voice Evaluation
Therapy Planning and the IEPC
Therapy

The following narrative is a case example of the application of the methods and concepts of voice therapy found in this book. It is of necessity an abbreviated account, providing only the high points of the treatment process. This, of course, represents our interpretation of a clinical program for this particular client. We have made periodic comments in the narrative in order to stress certain clinical concepts or procedures. We also wish to reiterate the basic clinical concept set forth early in this book, that therapy with a vocal behavior is essentially no different from therapy with an articulation behavior. The basic therapy procedures remain the same; the only difference is the behavior being modified.

The Referral and Voice Evaluation

Pat is a speech clinician in a public school program in Michigan. She has worked in the schools for 20 years and has her professional routine very well established: scheduling children for therapy, writing reports, setting aside time for evaluations, writing reports, participating in IEPCs, writing reports, and, if there is time left, providing therapy and writing reports. Pat remembers the times when she spent more time in therapy than she did writing reports, but that is history. Evaluations and therapy are now deeply involved in audits, accountability, records, and such. This is not all bad, Pat admits, but perhaps it has gone a bit too far. Yes, we should all be accountable for our therapy but we should be given adequate time to do it and we should have objective criteria to evaluate our clinical progress. However, things get a bit confused when attempts are made to "objectify" communicative behaviors such as stuttering and voice disorders, especially when you have to "label" the disorder and attempt to rate its "severity."

When Pat picked up her mail she found a Voice Checklist form on a child that was being referred by a teacher in one of the schools to which she provided clinical services. The referral was on a standard form used by the district where she worked. She looked over the form and found that the teacher had a referred a third grade boy by the name of Tim. The teacher had checked items indicating that Tim cannot be heard adequately while reciting, loses his voice during the day, and talks loud or shouts a great deal, and that his voice quality gets worse during the day and distracts from what he is saying.

Pat sent a letter to Tim's parents asking permission to examine him for a possible voice disorder. She carefully set forth in the letter

—NOTES—

all of the information required under PL 92–142. When the parents had signed the necessary forms, Pat scheduled a voice evaluation. She worked with Tim's teacher, who had made the referral, and scheduled a time for her evaluation. On the day of the evaluation she went to the classroom, got Tim, and took him to her clinical area, a small room the nurse uses when she visits the school.

> The professional clinician uses informal data collection to make some very important decisions or impressions. She can decide what category the disorder falls in, such as language or voice, or if the problem interferes with normal communication. She uses the informal data collection to help her focus on the problem at hand.

On the way to the room she talked to Tim in order to form some immediate impressions of his vocal production. His voice quality and pitch seemed to be the main problems. She could hear air escaping during his voicing but low pitched noise was also present in his voice. Pat had been trained to identify the acoustic characteristics of voice, and the best she could do with this voice was to classify it as a "hoarse" voice. She also noted that there were times when Tim tried to vocalize, such as with the word "gum," but produced a complete lack of phonation on the word. So she had two factors, a voice that was "hoarse" when there was vocalization but also periodic aphonia. She also felt that Tim's voice was too low in pitch for an 8 year old boy.

By the time they arrived at the therapy room, she had decided that Tim's voice problem could be acoustically classified as a hoarse voice with periodic aphonia and with a low pitch and insufficient loudness.

GENERAL DATA COLLECTION

> The clinician selects a collection of test instruments that will assist her in making objective assessments of a potential communication disorder. When the problem is unknown, the tests cover a wide variety of assessments. When the problem is isolated, such as with voice, the choice is to describe the behavior in as much detail as possible with the hope of finding both the cause and effect relationship and a therapy that is designed to meet the needs of the diagnosis.

When they were in the room and seated at the table, Pat took a copy of the Voice Behavior Profile Sheet (VBPS) and filled out the top of the form. Where it asked for an auditory classification for the voice problem she wrote in that the voice was hoarse; periodic aphonia was present; the pitch was too low; and the voice was too soft. She then continued her collection of general information by asking Tim about his voice: how he felt his voice sounded, if he ever had any problems getting people to understand him, and so forth. She took as much of a history as she could from Tim and then performed an oral-peripheral examination and other routine procedures in an evaluation. She entered her findings on the VBPS.

She had very little to enter on the VBPS from this general appraisal. There was nothing important set forth in the history and her observations of his performance and the oral-peripheral examination were not fruitful. About the only thing she could write on the VBPS was that he was cooperative but seemed a little hyperactive.

COMPETENCE/PERFORMANCE EVALUATION

Many clinicians prefer to evaluate behaviors rather than rely only on clinical judgments. It increases their objectivity and accuracy in diagnosing and reporting.

The next step in her evaluation was the competence/performance evaluation. She had Tim read one paragraph from a class book while standing and the next paragraph while seated. She watched carefully to see if his breathing was appropriate. She then had him stand and read a paragraph but start his reading by taking in a very deep breath. This time she noted that he pulled his stomach in and raised his shoulders when inhaling. She then decided to have him shout and when he took in a deep breath, his stomach went in and the shoulders went up again. She noted this on the VBPS along with the comment that this type of breathing did not occur except when he took a very deep breath or was speaking very loud. She also noted that he seemed to run out of air while speaking.

Her next task was to see how well Tim used his checking action during exhalation. She said to Tim, "I want you to make an 'ah' sound as long as you can but there cannot be any sound when you say the 'ah.' You open your mouth wide and exhale slowly. Watch me and I will show you how this is done." She showed Tim how to do this a couple of times and had him try it. The first and second trials were not correct but Tim caught on by the third trial. Now that Tim was ready to do this task, she had him perform it three times and timed each effort. The average of the three trials was 34 seconds and she wrote this on the VBPS.

It was now time to test Tim's ability to approximate his vocal folds. The first test was to see how well Tim could open and close the folds, starting with the vocal folds open. Her instructions to Tim were, "I want you to do a very slow laugh for me. Listen to me and then you try it: 'Hhhaaahhhaaa.' When you try it, remember not to stop between sounds, just keep laughing slowly." After a couple of trials Tim could do it. However, the movement from nonvoicing to voicing was not smooth and the vocal tone seemed to break up as the phonation started. She wrote this on the VBPS along with a note that Tim seemed to have some difficulty in doing this. She also noted that the vocal tone seemed to break up, containing both low pitched noise and the sound of air escaping.

In order to check Tim's ability to open the vocal folds from the closed position to the voicing position, she had Tim perform a series of "ah" sounds, each of which was separated by a vocal stop, that is, stopping the vocalization but keeping the vocal folds closed. Again, she demonstrated this for Tim and then had him try it until he could perform the task. When he was able to perform the task, she noted that he had a lot of trouble getting his voice started when coming out of the stop position. This was evident in his slow and labored productions. She noted this on the evaluation form.

The next check had to do with the type of movement of Tim's vocal folds during phonation. If the vocal folds moved together in a synchronous manner, a clear vocal tone would be present, but if the folds were either not closing appropriately or vibrating at different frequencies, the tone would be distorted. She had Tim produce a vocalized "ah" as long as he could. She timed three productions and took an average that amounted to 14 seconds. This large difference between voiced and unvoiced productions was noted on the VBPS along with comments about the presence of high and low pitched noise accompanying the vocal tone.

The next task concerned the vibration of the vocal folds and consisted of timing Tim's production of an [s] and a [z] sound. She gave Tim three trials with each sound and took the average time. The time for the [s] sound was 33 seconds, whereas the time for the [z] sound was 12 seconds. Pat noted these times on the VBPS. These performances agreed with the discrepancy found on the schwa vowel productions.

The last task directed to the mode of vocal fold vibration was to evaluate the stability or consistency of the mode of vibration. Pat asked Tim if he and his family had gone on a vacation last summer. He said that they had gone to visit Washington, D.C. She asked him to tell her about the vacation. As he told her his experiences, she listened carefully to the voice quality. It changed from time to time as he talked, going from what she had decided was "hoarse" to a whisper. The voice faded away toward the end of each phrase and also when he was speaking softly. Pat noted on the evaluation form that the mode of vibration changed over time, changing from approximated and vibrating folds to separated and nonvibrating folds at random intervals in Tim's speech.

> In addition to voice, the larynx has two other important independent responsibilities. The intrinsic muscles of the larynx, through unique muscular settings, provide the vocal tone with pitch and with loudness, each of which is independent of the other.

The next three tasks Pat tested were directed at Tim's ability to make tension adjustments in the internal muscles in the larynx. The first task concerned Tim's pitch range and the stability of the vocal tones. She had Tim prolong a schwa vowel at his lowest pitch, his highest pitch, and at his "normal" pitch. She timed each of the three productions and entered the times on the form. She also noted that the duration of the highest pitch sound was considerably longer than the other two productions. Her final note here was that both Tim's "normal" pitch and his lowest pitch were very low considering his age and size.

Pat next evaluated Tim's ability to "slide" his pitch from low to high and from high to low. She had him start vocalizing a schwa vowel at his lowest pitch and then slide upward to his highest pitch. She noticed that there were some sections of the pitch slide that were missing; that is, there was no tone produced. When the process was reversed, starting with the highest pitch and sliding to the lowest, Tim had even more difficulty in maintaining voice, with large sections of the slide not voiced. Pat noted these periods of aphonia on the form and stated that they occurred more frequently on the falling slide.

Having completed her evaluation of internal laryngeal adjustments that result in pitch changes, Pat began the evaluation of adjustments that result in loudness changes. She first measured the duration of schwa vowels at Tim's normal loudness, his softest vocal production, and his loudest voice. She noted on the VBPS that the longest duration was associated with the loudest production of the vowel. She also made a note that the pitch of his loudest production was higher than the other productions.

The next step in evaluating Tim's laryngeal adjustments associated with loudness of the voice was to have Tim start with a soft production of the vowel and then gradually increase the loudness until he was producing it at his loudest level. She then reversed the process, having Tim go from a loud production to a soft one. Pat observed that the

—NOTES—

shift in loudness was not smooth, particularly when Tim started with his loud voice and then made it soft. He had great difficulty maintaining his voice production during the task, and this information was entered on the form.

> The independence of pitch and loudness behaviors is best tested when the client is asked to change both.

It was now time to check the interactions of the laryngeal adjustments that control pitch and loudness. There were a number of tasks associated with this part of the evaluation, but Pat felt they were necessary, since there did seem to be some problems associated with Tim's performance on both the independent pitch and loudness evaluations. If there were problems with independent action, there might be even greater problems when the two behaviors were interdependent, so she had Tim perform the series of behaviors. In these tasks, pitch and loudness were combined in many ways to see how well they performed in concert. Pat noticed that as the pitch was raised the voice also became louder and that the vibrational mode of the vocal folds seemed to become more efficient. Tim had most of his problems when the voice was soft and the pitch was low.

The last step in the competence/performance evaluation was to have Tim perform a series of exercises that tested the speed of closure of the nasopharyngeal port and the efficiency of that closure. The exercises consisted of combinations of and consonants that, when produced, would reflect inadequate speed of closure or incomplete closure. Tim performed all of the exercises to Pat's satisfaction and she noted this on the form.

> Many detailed evaluations cannot be completed in one clinical session. In addition, if the voice becomes fatigued, the data collected will not be valid.

There was not time to continue the evaluation, so Pat sent Tim back to his class. This was an appropriate time to break up the evaluation, since Tim was becoming fatigued and his voice was growing weaker. After Tim left, Pat reviewed her findings and attempted to synthesize them in her mind. First, Tim had a problem with vocal fold approximation; the folds did not approximate but remained slightly open during phonation. However, when the pitch of the voice went up or the voice was made louder, the efficiency of the vocal fold closure increased.

The second basic finding was that the vocal folds vibrated in an asynchronous mode, with the two folds vibrating at different frequencies. In addition, there were many periods when the vocal folds just did not vibrate when they should have, thus producing aphonia. With these problems of closure and mode of vibration Pat was not surprised that there were also problems with pitch and loudness. Since the pitch was too low, it would seem to indicate that there was added mass on one or both of the folds. If there was added mass on one fold, this would account for the asynchronous mode of vibration.

The cause of the vocal problem was beginning to take on some form for Pat. If the added mass was on the edge of one vocal fold, there could not be good approximation for phonation and the phonation would be very inefficient. This would explain the time difference between the "exhaled" sounds whose duration was dependent on checking action and phonated sounds whose duration depends on the efficiency of the vibrations of the vocal folds. Pat concluded from the competence/performance evaluation that there probably was a growth on the vocal folds that was interfering with the normal vocal fold phonatory functions. She also noted that the teacher had reported that Tim shouted a great deal and that his voice became progressively worse during the day.

INTEGRATED VOICE ANALYSIS

> In a thorough evaluation, impressions formed in evaluating individual behaviors are placed into perspective by evaluating the integrated behavioral function, connected speech.

The following week Pat saw Tim again. She saw him late in the day so she could evaluate his voice when it was at its weakest. This was the time to listen carefully to Tim's vocal production and see if there was a relationship between her findings on the competence/performance evaluation and his actual vocal production and note the findings on the Integrated Voice Analysis section of the VBPS. Pat sat and talked with Tim about his vacation to Washington, D.C., his hobbies, his pets, and other topics that were neutral and nonthreatening. Pat listened and observed carefully. There were no problems with breathing or checking action so she left the first two cells on the analysis form empty. She then focused on the vocal fold approximation as reflected in the voice quality. Pat could hear air escaping during the phonation so she knew there was inadequate approximation of the folds. She was also aware of periods of aphonia when the folds were not vibrating so she entered *Ai* on the form, indicating the inadequate closure. Pat also noted that Tim used a hard vocal onset to initiate phonation. This abusive behavior did not occur consistently but Pat felt it was a factor that should be dealt with so she also entered an *Ho* on the form.

She next focused on the mode of vibration of the folds. Pat knew that a person could have inadequate closure and yet have normal vibrations of the folds, as with a slightly "breathy" voice, but this was not what she heard from Tim. Tim's voice quality contained both high and low frequency noise, the sound of air escaping, and a low rattling or rumbling sound. It was very difficult for her to determine the actual pitch of Tim's voice because of the "noise" factors. The voice was never produced clearly, so Pat entered an $S-$ in the appropriate cell on the form.

Pat now concentrated on Tim's pitch and loudness. Even though it was difficult to establish a true pitch for Tim, Pat's overall impression was that the pitch was too low for a child Tim's age. She entered a $P-$ in the pitch cell. She also entered a $L-$ in the loudness cell, since Tim's voice was difficult to hear except when he was shouting. When Pat attended to Tim's general vocal prosody, she felt it was restricted, with inadequate pitch and loudness variations. She noted this on the form by entering a $Pr-$ on the form. The final task in the integrated voice analysis was to listen for nasal resonance. She did not detect any deviancy in resonance so she left the cell empty.

ENVIRONMENTAL GUIDANCE TESTING

> Vocal pedigogy has taught us that the placement, projection, and imagery of the voice often changes the output. A behavioral voice evaluation must consider the potential effects these concepts might have on the voice production.

Having completed this section of the voice evaluation Pat moved into the final testing phase, environmental guidance of vocal behaviors. This part of the evaluation was to check to see how Tim responded to environmental manipulation of various vocal behaviors. Pat asked Tim to step away from the table about 5 feet and count from one to five, loud enough so she could hear. When he had completed this, she asked him to step away even farther, about 10 feet, and repeat the exercise. She noticed that when Tim stepped away he talked louder to compensate for the distance and when he talked even louder, his pitch went up and the voice became clearer. This was verification of her findings in the competence/performance evaluation. She then had Tim come back to the table and sit across from her. She took her note pad and held it between them but about a foot higher than Tim's head. She then told him to count from one to five but to "talk over the pad of paper." Tim tilted his head back a bit and counted but there was no difference in his voice. Pat lowered the pad to just off the top of the table and told Tim to talk "under" the pad. This time Tim lowered his head to count but again there was no difference in his voice.

The next task listed on the form consisted of creating excess tension in the individual and then having him speak. She told Tim to grab hold of the seat of the chair he was sitting in and try to lift himself up and to say a long "ah" while he was doing this. When he tried to lift the seat of the chair and vocalize the sound, the voice was clearer. She made a note of this and went on the next item. She had him relax in his chair and worked to make him as relaxed as possible in the clinical environment. When she noticed that he was a bit more relaxed, she asked him to make a long "ah" sound. When he made it she detected that the voice quality was worse than his normal voice, containing more breathiness and hoarseness. She wrote her observations on the form and moved to the last item. She asked Tim to look at the ceiling directly over his head and say a long "ah" sound. When he did this the vocal tone improved. When she had him prolong a tone while looking down at his chest, the tonal quality deteriorated. These observations were noted and she took Tim back to his class.

Therapy Planning and the IEPC

Pat now reviewed all her data. Her judgments of Tim's voice in the integrated voice analysis fit in with her findings in the competence/performance evaluation. Further, the environmental guidance portion of the evaluation had also indicated that if the tension in the folds was increased or the subglottal air pressure was increased, the force of the vibration was increased and this compensated for the faulty closure. She was now convinced that the behavioral problems with vocal fold approximation and vibrational mode, along with pitch and loudness problems, were the result of some growth on the vocal folds. However, this was only a hunch on her part, since she could not view the vocal folds, and even if she were able to see them, she was not qualified to make such a diagnosis. Therefore, Pat made the necessary arrangements to have Tim examined by a physician. She was fortunate in that her district had consulting physicians who would perform such examinations. The examination was cleared with Tim's parents and the physician did an examination of Tim's vocal folds. Pat prepared a statement for the physician stating her findings and that she suspected some sort of growth or added mass on the vocal folds.

> Reporting to a physician a list of behaviors that are consistent with vocal nodes is better than a referral that does not include objective information. The physician is apt to be more thorough in his evaluation with this information in mind.

The physician's report to Pat indicated that Tim did indeed have a vocal nodule on the left vocal fold and that the folds themselves were irritated and swollen. He also reported that Tim had an allergy that created problems of nasal drainage, mouth breathing, and clearing of the throat. The physician had prescribed medication to deal with the allergy.

Having gathered all of the necessary data, Pat set about preparing her presentation to Tim's parents at the IEPC meeting. She organized her findings in such a way that the parents would be able to understand what she did and why she did it. She then prepared a presentation to explain why vocal nodes develop, what they lead to, and what alternatives the parents have in terms of dealing with the problem.

> Preparation for effective communication with the parent is critical! The professional clinician should have objective data to support her recommendations, but she also must be able to communicate her findings and recommendations in a manner that is easily understood by the parents and other professionals. Professional jargon should be avoided.

In preparation of the IEPC meeting, Pat organized her therapy program for Tim. She recognized that there was a pathologic condition here that was interfering with Tim's ability to produce normal voice. The vocal folds would not be able to approximate normally until the added mass, the vocal node, was eliminated. The clinical question the parents would have to deal with was whether to have the node surgically removed or to go the route of therapy to remove the vocal abuse, which would in turn eliminate the vocal node. Her first clinical goal was to determine all those vocal behaviors that contributed to the vocal abuse. Her voice evaluation had pointed out two major sources of abuse, excessive shouting and improper breathing for loud speaking, which introduced tension into the laryngeal system. The physician had also suggested other behaviors, such as mouth breathing, which lead to a drying effect on the vocal folds, and throat clearing, which irritated the vocal folds. The medication should relieve the problem of mouth breathing and throat clearing, but the vocal abuse resulting from excessive shouting and improper breathing remained. Pat, in considering the excessive shouting, also recognized that according to the competence/performance evaluation data Tim did not have good independent functions of loudness and pitch. This meant that when Tim talked louder or shouted, the pitch would go up, a serious contributing factor to vocal abuse. So, in addition to reducing the amount of shouting, therapy should also have as a goal, the maintaining of normal pitch with increased loudness.

It was obvious to Pat that Tim was not motivated for therapy. His voice had not been creating problems for him, and only for his parents in terms of the aesthetic quality of his voice. Therefore, if Tim was not motivated to change his vocal habits, it would not be possible to eliminate all shouting, particularly in situations like on the playground or in the gymnasium. Therefore, it became crucial to attempt not only to reduce the amount of shouting but also to teach Tim a way to shout that was not harmful to the vocal folds. Pat's therapy program consisted of elimination of vocal abuse from incorrect breathing patterns and improper pitch level while talking loud. She also planned to reduce the amount of shouting by Tim. Other factors such as coughing and throat clearing would also be eliminated through the medication the physician had prescribed. Pat's therapy was planned in two stages. The first stage would be the removal of as many abusing behaviors as possible. The effects of this on the vocal node would be monitored by the physician. If this therapy program was successful and the node was absorbed, another evaluation would be made to see if further therapy was indicated.

At the IEPC meeting, Tim's parents were quite concerned about the vocal node and agreed that he could have therapy. Pat explained the concept of vocal abuse and how she would set up a therapy program that would eliminate many abusive behaviors and introduce new, nonabusive vocal behaviors. She also asked if the parents would be willing to participate in a home program. After she explained what she would expect them to do, they agreed to work with Pat by carrying out a program in the home. Pat was now ready to start her therapy with Tim.

> Therapy planning is critical to success. When data obtained in the evaluation provides behavioral objectives in a sequential fashion, much of the planning is already completed. However, the clinician must recognize that although some behaviors are easily modified, others will be difficult or even impossible to modify.

Pat had a number of things that she needed to teach Tim, such as how to breath without raising his shoulders, how to increase his loudness without raising his pitch, and how to reduce the amount of shouting he was doing. This last item would have to be worked out with his teacher and his parents, but there would have to be some cooperation on Tim's part. Pat first had to deal with Tim's lack of motivation to work on his speech. His speech did not bother him and the other children in his classes thought it was "interesting" or "cute" to talk that way. Thus, Pat had to create motivation in Tim. She did not feel she could create motivation by talking to him about the serious consequences of this problem. If the "cognitive" approach was out, what was left? Pat only had one way to deal with Tim's lack of motivation: Find some sort of reward that he wanted so much he would work hard to get it.

Therapy

Pat started Tim in therapy on an individual basis, seeing him twice a week for 10 minute sessions. The competence/performance evaluation indicated that the first behavior she should work on was proper breathing. Her clinical approach was based on the Clinical Interaction Model (CIM), so she considered how she would teach proper breathing: by modeling it, giving Tim information about it, guiding him to it, or using a combination of the three factors. She decided that she would first explain a little bit about breathing to Tim, especially how the abdomen should protrude during deep inhalation for loud speech, and then she would demonstrate it for him. She would use physical guidance when Tim attempted to breath deeply, holding his shoulders down to prevent clavicular breathing from occurring. The reward for good performance would be a poker chip, and Tim would be allowed to save them until the end of the session and then purchase a back-up reward from a box of rewards Pat had. Later in therapy there would be a clinical penalty in the form of taking a chip back, but Tim had to learn the new behavior before he could be penalized for the old behavior. If he was going to avoid the improper breathing in order to avoid the penalty, he needed to know how to breathe properly!

Pat was now ready to start Tim in therapy. The first clinical step was to explain the behavior change goal to Tim. She told him, "You have to learn a new way to take in a deep breath. When you do it now, you pull in your stomach and raise your shoulders. This hurts the little bands in your throat that you make sound with. I am going to ask you to take a deep breath in a minute and I want you to try to let your stomach go out. You will be thinking about your stomach so I am going to hold my hands on your shoulders to remind you to keep them down. Watch me while I take in a deep breath. (Pat models the behavior.) Did you notice that my stomach went out just a little bit when I took in the deep breath? And, did you notice that my shoulders did not rise? Watch me again. (Models again.) Now, I want you to take in a deep breath just like I did."

Tim stood up and took in a deep breath, sucking in his stomach and raising his shoulders a bit. Pat noted that even though the behavior was not correct, Tim was paying attention and trying. She said, "That

—NOTES—

wasn't too bad, Tim." This ended the first transaction on a bit of a positive note, a very small reward. The reward was more for his attention and attempt to perform the behavior than the actual production. She would have to repeat the task in the second clinical transaction but change her stimulus because Tim's performance indicated that he had not quite understood what he was expected to do.

Pat decided to repeat the model but add a bit more information for Tim. She said to Tim, "Let me show you again and you watch my stomach go out a little bit. And put your hand on my shoulder so you can feel that my shoulders do not go up. See how my chest and stomach go in and out together when I breath. Now, let's see if you can do that." This time she held Tim's shoulders down with more force. When Tim took in a deep breath his stomach came out a bit and Pat could feel less of an attempt to raise the shoulders. The behavior was much better. She told Tim that he did a very good job and she gave him a poker chip. The second transaction was successful.

> Rewards are vital to effective and efficient therapy. The major problem is trying to figure out an appropriate reward for each client in each clinical setting. The Token Economy solves these problems by providing each client with a "token" reward that can then be converted into a meaningful reward at the end of the therapy session.

Tim looked at the chip, a bit confused as to why he had it. Pat started the third transaction but first gave Tim information about the chip. She explained to him, "The chip you have is just like money; you can buy things with it. Look in this box and you can see a lot of little things that you can buy. Each one has a price on it; it tells you how many chips you need to buy it. You will get more chips as we practice the new way of breathing. Every time you do it right, I will give you a chip, and then when we are finished today, you can pick out what you want from the box. You just have to remember that you have to have enough chips to buy what you want." When Pat was finished explaining the token economy she said, "Tim, how do you earn chips?" He thought for a second and then said, "I get one when I breathe right." Pat knew that he understood so she smiled (another form of reward) and told him that he was correct. The third transaction was also concluded with a reward.

The fourth transaction started with Pat asking Tim if he could breathe right without being shown the model. She said, "I wonder if you can breathe right and get a chip without my showing you how. I will hold your shoulders down but that is all I am going to do. Show me how you can do it." Tim stood up and, with Pat barely touching his shoulders, took in a deep breath without raising the shoulders and with the stomach protruding. Pat told Tim how well he did and gave him a chip. Pat was now well on her way to becoming an S + for Tim, cuing the new behavior to occur because of the reward.

Transactions that followed focused on making the new breathing pattern more natural and having it occur without any modeling, information, or guidance from Pat. By the end of this session Tim could take in a deep breath normally. He had earned 13 chips, which he used to buy something from Pat's box of rewards.

> Although the token reward may first lack meaning for the client, as soon as it is associated with buying a back-up reward, it takes on real value. The back-up reward is very important, since each client gets to choose what ever he wants, or can afford, from a variety of items the clinician has available. When a client learns that he is going to be rewarded for performing a behavior and then performs that behavior in order to get the reward, this is referred to as approach motivation.

As this clinical goal was being accomplished, Pat added a second component to her therapy to attempt to minimize the amount and type of shouting that Tim was doing. She felt that there was no possible way she would be able to eliminate Tim's shouting, since almost all boys shout as part of their normal routine, but she could eliminate some of it and change the type of shouting that remained. First of all she would change the existing shouting behavior by making the vocal loudness independent of the pitch. She would start by having Tim count up to five at his normal loudness and pitch level. She would then have him count again, a little louder but at the same pitch. She would repeat this until Tim could talk quite loud without raising his pitch. At the same time she would expect Tim to breathe correctly as he was taking in a deep breath for the louder talking.

Pat started this series of transactions by giving Tim a complex stimulus of modeling, information about loudness and pitch, and gestural guidance in the form of hand gestures associated with vocal loudness and pitch. Motioning toward herself meant to increase the loudness, motioning away meant to decrease the loudness, pointing up meant to raise the pitch, and pointing down meant to lower the pitch. During each succeeding transaction Pat would ask Tim to count louder. As the loudness increased there was a tendency for the pitch to go up, so she would point down while Tim was counting. Each time he was successful she would give him a chip. As the loudness of the counting increased, Tim's shoulders began to move slightly. On the next transaction

—NOTES—

Pat said to Tim, "Your shoulders are moving just a bit so I will put my hand on your shoulders to remind you not to move them. Now, count again and make it just a bit louder but don't let your pitch go up." Tim counted again and this time he did not raise his shoulders. Pat praised him and gave him another token. By the end of the session Tim could talk quite loud without raising his pitch. At the end of the session he bought something from Pat's box of rewards. She was a solid S+ now. The rewarded behaviors occurred naturally whenever she was present.

> Whenever a person or an environment is associated with a reward, that person or environment becomes a positive stimulus. It cues or prompts whatever behavior has been rewarded to occur so the person can receive another reward. When clients come into a therapy room, their new behaviors are cued or prompted by the room and the clinician. When a client is performing a behavior in order to achieve a reward, it is referred to as approach motivation. However, when the client is out of this environment, the behaviors are no longer cued or prompted.

After several sessions Pat changed the rules of the token economy. She explained the rule changes to Tim, saying, "From now on, Tim, when you talk loud and your breathing and pitch are good, I will give you a chip. But if you raise your shoulders while breathing or raise your pitch when talking loud, I will take back a chip. Do it right and you get a token; do it wrong and you lose one." Pat knew that Tim could do the behaviors correctly if he would just remember to perform them. The penalty was a way to remind him, a way to make sure he would avoid breathing incorrectly or raising his pitch. During the first four transactions Pat had Tim counting up to fifteen. He had to stop several times and take breaths in order to count that high while talking very loud. He forgot about his breathing and pitch in the third transaction so Pat took back a chip. Pat immediately became an S— for the incorrect behaviors of raising the shoulders and the pitch. Tim was upset that he lost a chip. On the next transaction Tim was very careful not to breathe wrong or let the pitch go up. He got a chip for that performance and then Pat changed her stimulus to asking Tim questions about his favorite game, baseball. Tim had to answer in a loud voice without allowing his pitch to go up and every time he spoke this way he received another chip. However, Tim became very involved in telling Pat about his game a week ago and forgot about his behaviors. Pat took another chip. Tim was very careful for the rest of the session.

Negative learning or learning to avoid a penalty is a very strong form of learning. Things associated with negative learning situations assume the role of a negative stimulus. They cue or prompt a behavior *not* to occur. A red traffic light is an S − , prompting drivers not to continue driving but to stop. If a driver does not pay attention to the S − , a penalty will occur, such as an accident or a traffic ticket. When a client is attempting to avoid a penalty by not performing a specific behavior, it is referred to as avoidance motivation.

It was now time to test the new behaviors outside of the therapy room. Pat talked to Tim's teacher about how she could help Tim use the new behaviors in the classroom. The teacher agreed to help, so Pat set up a form of token economy with the teacher. First, if Tim talked loud at a normal pitch in a situation in which he would have normally shouted, the teacher was to make a note of this so Tim could get a chip when he went to therapy. Second, if Tim did shout, but it was at a lower pitch, a note would be made for another chip. Finally, if Tim shouted with his old voice, a note would be made so that Pat could take a token away at the time the notes from the teacher were reviewed. The teacher was now taking on the roles of an S + for the new behaviors and an S − for the old behaviors. Pat kept careful track of the teacher's comments and determined that the token economy was working. The rewarded behaviors were increasing in frequency of occurrence, whereas the penalized behavior of shouting at a high pitch was happening less. She reviewed the teacher's comments with Tim and praised him for his performance. As therapy was progressing, Tim's voice quality was improving, as there was less abuse of the vocal folds.

Generalization of newly learned behaviors to the client's outside environments is the most difficult phase of therapy, since the clinician cannot be present to remind the client to perform the newly acquired behavioral skill. Therefore, the clinician must establish other S + and S − in the client's environments, both in the school and in the home. These stimulus roles are established by associating an individual with either a reward (S +) or a penalty (S −). In order to maintain these stimulus roles, the individual must be consistent in his responses and continue them over a period of time. Once the reward or penalty is no longer presented, the individual loses the stimulus role and becomes neutral, an S0.

As these behaviors were being generalized into Tim's school environment, Pat moved on to the next behavior change goal, easy vocal onset. The integrated voice analysis indicated that Tim initiated many of his vocalizations from a closed position of the vocal folds, a hard vocal onset. When Tim attempted to produce a vowel sound for Pat, he would move abruptly from the closed position of the folds to vocalizing the sound. Pat decided to use the [h] sound to teach Tim easy vocal onset. In the first transaction of this new behavioral goal, Pat explained to Tim, "When we say a vowel, like *a, e, i, o,* or *u,* we want to 'slide' into the sound gradually. We don't want to start when we are holding our breath. Let me show you how we can start 'hard' when we are holding our breath (demonstrates hard vocal onset on a vowel). Now I will start 'easy,' sliding into the sound (demonstrates easy vocal onset introducing the vowel with a very short [h] sound). Can you hear that they are different?" Tim responded that he could not hear a difference, so Pat had to repeat the transaction. However, this time she told Tim what to listen for and exaggerated the [h] when she modeled the two sounds. This time Tim said he could hear the difference, Pat moved to the next step, the introduction of the [h] to Tim as a means of achieving easy vocal onset. She told him that he could slide into the sound if he would use the [h] sound, and she modeled the easy vocal onset on the vowel *a,* exaggerating the duration of the [h] and slowing the shift to the vowel. When Tim attempted to imitate the model it went rather well, and Pat rewarded him with a chip. The transactions that followed were focused on making sure Tim could consistently produce the easy vocal onset using the [h] sound.

Pat then decided it was time to put Tim in a shaping group for therapy. She put him in a group with three other children, two of whom had articulation problems and the third child a stuttering problem. When she introduced Tim to the group she had him demonstrate what he was working on. She then had each of the other children demonstrate what they were working on. From this point on, the group members began to determine how well Tim was doing on his behavior and they would reward him with the group reward, chips. The group concentrated on shortening the duration of Tim's [h] sound, shaping the behavior to the correct form of easy onset.

> Group therapy is a valuable clinical tool for the school clinician. It not only provides a means of social practice for new speech behaviors, it gives the clinician an extremely strong reward or penalty (peer opinion) and creates a number of conditioned stimuli in the school setting; that is, each member of the group becomes both an S+ and an S− to the other members of the group. They then assist in the carry-over of the new behavior to the school environment.

Tim's vocal behavior in school had changed drastically. The amount of shouting had been reduced and the shouting that remained

—NOTES—

was at a normal pitch, reducing the amount of abuse on the vocal folds. As Tim began to use the easy vocal onset even more abuse was eliminated. Pat felt that swelling of the vocal folds must be decreasing, since Tim could produce a clearer tone and there seemed to be less aphonia. At this point Pat repeated the competence/performance evaluation and the integrated voice analysis. She found that Tim's breathing was now normal; he could approximate his folds better; there was very little noise in the vocal tone; the periods of aphonia had disappeared; the pitch was closer to normal for a boy his age; and the loudness of the vocal tone had increased.

Pat arranged a conference with Tim's mother and shared these findings with her. She also asked the mother if she would start a token economy in the home, rewarding Tim for his new speech behaviors and penalizing him for the old behaviors. The mother agreed and Pat set up the rules for a token economy, setting forth the behaviors to be rewarded and penalized, what the back-up rewards would be, how often the behaviors would be rewarded and so forth. Pat set into motion through this home program the mechanism for the parents to change their stimulus roles from that of an S0 to an S+ and an S−.

> A clinician might rely on the habit strength of the new vocal behaviors to carry over the new behaviors into the home environment, but this is an extremely inefficient process. If parental cooperation can be obtained, it is wiser to address the problem directly in the home. By establishing a home-based token economy, the generalization of the new behavior can be made more effective and efficient by creating new S+ and S− to cue or prompt the behaviors in that environment.

As therapy progressed, Tim's voice continued to improve. Pat was certain that the vocal node was getting smaller, but she needed some evidence to verify that her therapy program was effective. Therefore, she referred Tim back to the physician who had performed the original examination. The physician verified Pat's clinical data, reporting that the node had all but disappeared and the vocal folds appeared to be all but free of signs of vocal abuse. Pat continued the group therapy program for two more months and worked with the parents to stabilize the new behaviors in the home. The other members of Tim's shaping group continued to act as S+ for Tim as he would encounter them in school, and the parents, in their S+ role, cued the behaviors to occur in Tim's external environments.

When the reports from the parents, teachers, and other members of Tim's shaping group indicated that Tim was no longer using the abusive vocal behaviors, Pat revised his clinical schedule so that Tim was

—NOTES—

included in the shaping group only once a month. At this time Pat performed another voice evaluation on Tim. The physiological problem had been resolved, so it was now time to see if Tim could perform all of the vocal behaviors necessary for normal voice.

> If a medical or physiological condition can be remediated, it is necessary to evaluate the client after the change has been made to see how well he can now perform the various behaviors necessary for normal voice. If there still remains some behavioral problems, therapy should be continued until the behavior can be performed adequately. In another instance the effects of a medical or physiological condition may be only reduced, not eliminated. The re-examination is extremely vital in order to evaluate the behavioral performances once the interfering factor has been reduced or eliminated.

Pat's re-examination proved to be negative, both in terms of the competence/performance evaluation and the integrated voice analysis. Her findings were that Tim could now perform all vocal behaviors adequately and that his auditory vocal performance was normal. With this data in hand plus the reports on Tim's vocal performance from the parents, teachers, and members of Tim's shaping group, Pat scheduled another IEPC meeting to decertify Tim. Because Pat had included Tim's parents in the clinical process and they were aware of the progress Tim had made, they agreed that the vocal problem had been eliminated and the IEPC agreed to decertify Tim. He was subsequently dismissed from therapy.

The Voice Evaluation: Procedures and Rating Form

GENERAL DATA COLLECTION

1. Make a subjective auditory classification of the client's voice, that is, hoarse, harsh, breathy, pitch too high, voice too soft, nasal, and so on.
2. Collect a personal history and a history of vocal disorder.
3. Observe the client's general motor activities, with particular attention to fine motor skills. Note any unusual observations.
4. Test the client's hearing and perform an oral-peripheral examination, noting any unusual findings.

COMPETENCE/PERFORMANCE EVALUATION

1. Examine the client's mode of breathing. Note if opposition or clavicular breathing modes are present. Have client read while standing and while seated. Have the client read with normal breathing and with deep breaths. Converse with the client. Observe breathing patterns.
2. Determine the adequacy of checking action (breath control). Time the duration of an exhalation with the client "thinking" of the schwa vowel but not voicing it. Take the average of three trials. Also see Item 4.
3a. Determine the client's ability to approximate the vocal folds. Note the diadochokinetic rate of on/off voicing with easy vocal attack. Have the client produce as series of [hɑ] sounds, like a slow laugh.
3b. Determine the client's ability to open the vocal folds for phonation. Note the diadochokinetic rate of on/off voicing with hard vocal attack. Have the client produce a series of [ɑ] sounds, each separated by a vocal stop.
4a. Check the synchronization of the movements of the vocal folds. Have the client prolong a schwa vowel as long as he can. Measure the duration of the vowel. Compare your findings with the duration of the voiceless schwa produced in Item 2. Listen for the presence of "noise" in the vocal tone.
4b. Determine the mode of vocal fold vibration by measuring durations of prolonged [s] and [z] sounds. The duration of the [z] should be equal to or greater than the [s] owing to the vocal folds involvement in checking action. The production of a [z] that is in excess of [s] production could imply excessive vocal fold approximation, whereas shorter [z] production could imply inadequate vocal fold approximation.

—NOTES—

4c.   Determine the stability of the vocal fold vibration. Regardless of the degree of closure or the mode of vibration, the vocal folds should be consistent in their vibrations over time. Instability is apparent when the folds periodically shift in the degree of closure or their mode of vibration. Have the client tell a story, recount a vacation, or talk about any topic that will elicit speech. If there are changes in vocal tone, note where and when they occur.

5a.   Investigate the client's vocal duration at various pitch levels. Have the client prolong a schwa sound at his normal pitch, his highest pitch, and his lowest pitch. Note the duration of each production. The pitch in each attempt should be stable, and there should be little if any difference in duration.

5b.   Check the client's ability to change pitch in a smooth fashion. Have the client vocalize a schwa vowel at his lowest pitch and then slide the tone to his highest pitch. Reverse the procedure, starting with the highest pitch. Note any breaks in the pitch or missing segments.

6a.   Investigate the client's vocal duration at various loudness levels. Have the client prolong a schwa sound at an average loudness level, at his softest level, and at his loudest level. Note the duration of each production. The loudness in each attempt should be stable, and there should be little if any difference in duration.

6b.   Check the client's ability to change loudness in a smooth fashion. Have the client vocalize a schwa vowel at his softest level and then slide the tone to his loudest. Reverse the procedure, starting with the loudest production. Note any breaks in the loudness change.

7.   Determine the adequacy in laryngeal adjustments for pitch and loudness. Have the client perform the following tasks and make note of observable changes in approximation, synchronization, and the ability of pitch and loudness changes to occur independent of one another. Have the client produce the schwa vowel under the following conditions:
   a.   High pitch/loud voice
   b.   High pitch/soft voice
   c.   Low pitch/loud voice
   d.   Low pitch/soft voice
   e.   Low pitch ascending to high pitch (soft voice)
   f.   Low pitch ascending to high pitch (loud voice)
   g.   High pitch descending to low pitch (loud voice)
   h.   High pitch descending to low pitch (soft voice)
   i.   Soft voice increasing to loud voice (low pitch)
   j.   Soft voice increasing to loud voice (high pitch)
   k.   Loud voice descending to soft voice (high pitch)
   l.   Loud voice descending to soft voice (low pitch)

8.   Evaluate the competence of the nasopharyngeal port action. Have the client perform the following tasks and note any problems the client might have in isolating the nasal resonator from the vocal system. Also note any problems the client might have in coordinating the palatal movements.
   a.   Have the client count from 60 to 70.
   b.   Have the client repeat the following as fast as possible:
      1.   [mpa, mpa, mpa, mpa]
      2.   [pam, pam, pam, pam]
      3.   [map, map, map, map]

c.   Have the client produce consonant-vowel and vowel-consonant combinations from the following:

[i]   [m]
[a]   [k]
[u]   [h]

d.   Have the client speak with exaggerated jaw opening.

INTEGRATED VOICE ANALYSIS

Engage the client in a conversation in which he does most of the talking such as his telling you a story. As he is talking evaluate the influence of the following behaviors in the ongoing speech. Rate the influence of each behavior according to the scale provided on the VBPS:
1. Breathing patterns
2. Checking action
3. Vocal fold approximation
4. Vocal fold mode of vibration
5. Pitch level
6. Loudness level
7. Prosody
8. Nasal resonance

ENVIRONMENTAL GUIDANCE OF VOCAL BEHAVIORS

Have the client perform the following tasks in order to test his vocal adjustments to environmental factors. Note any changes in breathing, checking action, vocal fold approximation, mode of vibration of the folds, pitch, loudness, prosody, or nasal resonance that occur.

1. Have the client speak to you loud enough for you to hear him as you increase the distance between you.
2. Have the client speak "over" and "under" a barrier held between you.
3. Have the client produce a schwa vowel with increased tension, such as trying to pick up his chair while he is sitting on it.
4. Have the client produce a schwa vowel while relaxed. Use a relaxation method presented in Appendix B.
5. Have the client produce a schwa vowel while looking at the ceiling over his head and while holding his chin against his chest.

—NOTES—

Voice Behavior Profile Sheet
W. R. Leith and R. G. Johnston

Client _____   Date _____

Clinician _____   Agency _____

General Data Collection

Initial classification _____

Findings from general appraisal _____

_____
_____
_____
_____
_____
_____

Competence/Performance Evaluation
Findings and Comments

1. Breathing patterns _____
_____
_____

2. Checking action _____
_____

3a, b. Vocal fold approximation _____
_____

4a, b, c. Vocal fold vibrational mode _____
_____

5a, b. Vocal pitch _____
_____

6a, b. Vocal loudness _____
_____

7. Pitch/loudness interaction _____
_____

8. Nasopharyngeal port adjustments _____
_____
_____

—NOTES—

Integrated Voice Analysis

Behavior	Rating	Codes
1. Breathing patterns	_____	Adequate, leave cell empty; incorrect pattern, Bp –.
2. Checking action	_____	Adequate, leave cell empty; inadequate, Ca –.
3. V F approximation	_____	Adequate, leave cell empty; inadequate, Ai; excessive, Ae; variable, Av; hard onset, Ho.
4. V F mode of vibration	_____	Synchronous, leave cell empty; asynchronous, S –; variable, Sv.
5. Pitch level	_____	Appropriate, leave cell empty; too high, P +; too low, P –.
6. Loudness level	_____	Appropriate, leave cell empty; too loud, L +; too soft, L –.
7. Prosody	_____	Appropriate, leave cell empty; too variable, Pr +; too restricted, Pr –.
8. Nasal resonance	_____	Appropriate, leave cell empty; excessive, N +; inadequate, N –.

Comments _____

_____

_____

_____

Environmental Guidance of Vocal Behaviors

Factor	Comments
Distance	_____
Barrier	_____
Tension	_____
Relaxation	_____
Extension/flexion	_____

Relaxation Techniques

General body tension usually manifests itself in an increase in tension in the larynx. With increased tension in the larynx, the behaviors necessary for normal vocal production are inhibited and this results in vocal changes. We have long recognized that localized tension in the larynx has an effect on vocal production. How many times have you heard someone say, "I had such a lump in my throat I could hardly talk." Usually this occurs after an emotional experience, such as seeing a very sad movie. When laryngeal tension becomes chronic (present all the time), it creates a problem, since it now interferes with vocal production over extended periods of time.

Physical body tension is characteristic of many clients who come for voice therapy. This tension can often be observed, especially in the strap muscles in the neck. With increased tension in the neck, there are several reasons why voice therapy may not be successful if the tension is allowed to persist. The most obvious reason is that the intrinsic muscles of the larynx are quite small in comparison to other muscles influencing laryngeal action, such as the strap muscles. When these larger muscles are tense they inhibit the delicate and subtle movements of the smaller intrinsic muscles, which are necessary for fine control over vocal production. Rather than starting out by searching for reasons for the tension, it is often clinically sound to eliminate the tension to determine if a positive change in the vocal behaviors will take place.

The client may learn the essence of relaxation in one session or less. Applying the relaxation outside of therapy requires careful planning, practice, and motivation. For the purposes of this book, we will provide two methods of relaxation proven to be effective for us. The first is a general form of relaxation termed *tension-relaxation contrast* and is used when the client is reporting overall tension during speaking. The second is a direct form of relaxation termed *pressure-point massage* and is used when the client is reporting specific tension (as in the neck area) during speaking.

TENSION-RELAXATION CONTRAST

A client who has a high level of general body tension that may be interfering with normal vocal production should be taught to contrast the different feelings associated with high and low levels of tension. Start with the client seated comfortably in a chair or lying on a mat. When you speak to the client, speak in a calm and assuring manner.

1. Start the procedure by asking the client to close his eyes and to breathe deeply and slowly.
2. Inform the client, "We are going to begin learning how to relax. Please try your best to do what I ask you to do. First, I would like you to tighten your

right hand, making a tight fist, and hold it for 5 seconds (count off the 5 seconds). Now let your hand go. Notice the difference between how your hand felt when it was tight and how it feels now that it is relaxed. Let's do that again, and as you change your hand from tight to relaxed, do it slowly and feel the tension leaving your hand. Now that we have practiced on your hand, we will proceed through your body by tensing and relaxing other parts. Let me know if you do not understand or if I'm going too fast. Ready?'' The amount of time you spend on this and other parts of the body will depend on your client's cooperation and motivation. You must make the judgment of when to move to the next body part based on your appraisal of the degree of relaxation achieved and what your relaxation goal is.

3. Continue through the body in the sequence listed below. Remember that with each muscle group the client is to tense the muscles to their maximum, hold the tension for 5 seconds, slowly release the tension, and compare the difference in the tense and the relaxed conditions.

4. The following muscle groups and order is suggested:

Right hand
Right arm
Left hand
Left arm
Neck and shoulders
Face
Chest
Back
Abdomen
Entire upper body
Buttocks
Thighs
Feet
Entire body

5. Complete the exercise by asking the client to sit or lie quietly for a short period of time. A period of 5 minutes would be ideal. When the quiet period is completed, complete the section of the competence/performance evaluation associated with relaxation or, if relaxation is part of the therapy program, proceed with therapy. Generalized tension may negatively influence various vocal behavior performances. A change in performance scores on the competence/performance evaluation may be evidence that the client would benefit from tension-relaxation contrast, and the procedure can then be incorporated into the therapy program.

PRESSURE-POINT MASSAGE

If a client does not have general, overall tension but rather localized tension in specific muscle groups, then pressure-point massage intervention may be used to overcome the tension problem. This intervention is particularly useful when the tension appears to be concentrated in the head or neck region, or both, particularly with the strap muscles. You must have the understanding and consent of the client before proceeding because you will use be using a "hands-on" approach.

—NOTES—

1. Start the procedure by explaining to the client that you are going to massage and put pressure on certain muscles. The procedure may cause some mild discomfort but that the discomfort is necessary to achieve the correct result.
2. Seat the client in a comfortable chair and position yourself behind the chair. The client may close his eyes if he prefers.
3. Place the palm of your hand on top of the client's head and push down on the head as if you were pushing the head into the neck. Hold this push for 5 seconds, slowly rotating the head left then right. Release the head pressure quickly and call the client's attention to the release of tension as you stop pushing and he stops resisting the push. Tell him that this is the essence of the procedure: You will push hard on several spots on the body and he will resist. When you release the pressure and he stops resisting he is to feel the difference between the two conditions and the release of tension. The following pressure points can be massaged:

     Top of the head
     Forehead
     Temples
     Eyelids
     Upper bridge of the nose
     Temporal mandibular joint
     Mastoid bone
     Just lateral to the thyroid notch
     Just superior to the sternum
     Base of the neck
4. The procedure should be repeated with additional pressure up to the point at which the client experiences mild discomfort. When the pressure is released, discuss with the client the relief he feels as the muscles stop resisting and relax. After two presentations of the technique to the various points the following procedure is useful.
5. Cup the client's head under his chin and tell him, "I am going to hold your head up for you. As I massage your neck with my other hand, let your head rest in my hand and I will hold it for you."
6. After the client has relinquished muscular control of his head to your hand, gently roll the client's head back and forth. After you have held and rotated the head for about 1 minute, move the head back up into the erect position and slowly relinquish control back to the client.
7. Pressure-point massage therapy essentially attempts to relax specific muscle groups or body regions. Upon completion of the exercise, complete the section of the competence/performance evaluation associated with relaxation or, if relaxation is part of your therapy program, proceed with therapy.

Hygiene of the Voice

Hygiene is essentially preventative medicine. Vocal hygiene then means vocal practices that are healthy; vocal behaviors that do not injure or abuse the larynx. Any program designed to avoid or eliminate vocal abuse or misuse must take into account our understanding of laryngeal anatomy and physiology and how the vocal system works. Because the human larynx is a biological valve, its major purpose is to keep foreign matter out of the lungs. It also serves to expel foreign matter from the lungs and upper airway. Behaviors such as throat clearing, coughing, sneezing, grunting, lifting, bowel movement, and holding the breath are necessary biological uses of the larynx. Add to the list reflexive vocal behaviors such as crying and we have a long list of behaviors for which vocal hygiene can be compromised; that is, the vocal system abused or misused. This is in addition to the improper use of the voice during speaking or singing. It is important to take time to explain to our clients of all ages how the vocal mechanism works and how it helps us do so many important things. When clients understand what important functions the system performs, why their voice problem exists, and the purpose of therapy, vocal hygiene becomes important and meaningful to them.

Voice care can be divided into three major categories: the identification and elimination of *vocal abuse*, the identification and elimination of *vocal misuse*, and the identification and elimination of *environmental factors* that are inconsistent with good vocal hygiene.

VOCAL ABUSE

Abuse of the vocal system is very common. Because there is no sensation of pain in the vocal folds, clients often do many abusive things to the vocal folds, not realizing that they are damaging them. Following are some behaviors that can lead to vocal abuse when used in combinations or when used to excess:

Yelling
Screaming
Throat clearing
Coughing
Crying
Talking using hard vocal onset

These behaviors are usually associated with the occurrence of a specific laryngeal behavior, that is, the vigorous compression of the vocal folds to seal off the outflow of air and then the sudden release of air usually driven at high pressure. The result of this explosive release of air is that the vocal folds, having been blown far apart by the high air pressure, come back together and close vigorously, eventually injuring each other. Contact ulcers, vocal swelling, or nodules are the common end result.

Therapy

The client should be counseled regarding proper use of the vocal folds. He should be shown how to use an easy vocal onset to approximate the vocal folds. The easy onset can then be associated with speaking loudly, clearing the throat, and other similar voluntary behaviors. Correct approximation of the vocal folds and the reduction of occurrences of vigorous vocal fold closure are basic to the elimination of vocal abuse. The client should also be helped, along with significant others, to identify when, where, and how often he uses the potentially abusive behaviors. Once identified, he should be helped to eliminate or modify the behaviors. One way to help him is through the use of "reminders." It is especially helpful for the child client to have his parents or significant others "remind" him when he clears his throat to do it the "better way," that is, with the easy onset you taught him in therapy. You might also have the child keep a logbook on how well he is using the easy onset or eliminating the abusive behaviors, but you will have to work carefully with him in order for him to use it satisfactorily.

Vocal rest can also be an effective tool. If the client is placed on short mandatory periods of *no talking or whispering*, the voice is given an opportunity to rest; that is, the tissue is given a short period to recover. But the abusive behaviors must be modified in order for the periods of rest to have any permanent effect. Client motivation is essential in this therapy. The use of pictures of vocal nodules and information about surgical removal of nodes may have a motivational influence on the client and increase his willingness to participate in the vocal hygiene program.

VOCAL MISUSE

Vocal misuse is different from vocal abuse but can have the same negative effect on the health of the vocal folds. When we talk about misuse of the voice, we are saying that the client is essentially using his voice incorrectly. In vocal abuse, the trauma to the vocal folds came from a variety of behaviors with the common theme of vigorous closure and high pressure opening of the vocal folds. However, in vocal misuse, the only source of irritation of the vocal folds is from the use (or misuse) of the voice. Some of the main sources of vocal misuse are

Talking
Singing
Using the incorrect pitch
Using "strange" voices

The theme that develops with these clients is one of excess. Too much talking, too much singing, too high a pitch, too low a pitch, and so forth. Singing presents a special problem, since singing demands more phonation time and less silent or pause time than talking. A problem with both talking and singing concerns the pitch of the voice. If the pitch is too high or too low, the intrinsic muscles that are involved with pitch adjustments are overworked, causing fatigue. Perhaps more significant is that when the natural pitch of the vocal folds is changed, either to too high or low, the vocal folds are forced to vibrate at an unnatural pitch. As was pointed out in Chapter 3, this creates stress on the vocal folds. Unnatural vocal fold vibration is also the basis of the "strange" voices that are often produced by children. Again, if this becomes excessive it can create problems with the vocal folds.

Therapy

For the excessive talker who is misusing his voice, we suggest a program of silent periods during the day. Just as the human body needs rest, so does the human voice. The client, along with significant others, can set up a reasonable performance contract that allows for talking and silence at prescribed times. If the voice problem does not improve, silent time needs to be increased. If the problem improves, adjustments in the talking and silent times can be made until the problem is neutralized.

If the client is singing too much, you must counsel him about his misuse of the voice and suggest he discuss this with the music teacher or his singing coach. You might establish the client's natural pitch using the four or five tone method (singing up four or five notes from the lowest note the person is able to maintain) and pass this information on to the music teacher or voice coach. These are professional people who will recognize if the client is singing outside his vocal range.

Perhaps the most important clinical step to take here is to determine the natural pitch level for the client who is misusing his voice. Forced vibration of the vocal folds at unnatural pitch levels creates problems. The main culprit is high pitch level associated with shouting or yelling. As the some individuals increae loudness, they also raise their pitch. The competence/performance evaluation tests the independence of pitch and loudness controls and, if they are indeed independent functions, a person should be able to speak loudly or even shout without raising the pitch. This independence of control should be included as part of your therapy program. This is an important part of your therapy for the cheerleaders in your schools who may be referred for therapy.

We should also mention the use of strange or "funny" voices that many children use for their entertainment value. Strange voices put considerable stress on the entire laryngeal structure. These vocal behaviors should be eliminated through counseling and the use of significant others to remind the client to not use the behavior.

ENVIRONMENTAL FACTORS

Vocal abuse may be the natural result of the larynx performing its biological function under adverse physiological conditions: irritants, allergies, and certain foods may result in excessive coughing, sneezing, and clearing the throat. If a client persistently clears his throat (more than 10 times per hour) or coughs and sneezes when an upper respiratory infection is not present, then we may need to turn our attention to the identification and elimination of the factor causing this abuse of the vocal folds. Because the client is receiving therapy for a vocal disorder, we assume that he has already been seen by a physician and that some evidence of vocal abuse exists. If you feel that there is a problem with the frequency of throat clearing and coughing, make a note of this for the physician the next time you send the child back for the physician's periodic evaluation of the vocal folds.

References and Recommended Readings

Aronson, A. (1980). *Clinical voice disorders: An interdisciplinary approach*. New York: Thieme-Stratton.

Berger, E. (1981). *Parents as partners in education*. St. Louis: C. V. Mosby.

Boone, D. (1977). *The voice and voice therapy*. Englewood Cliffs, NJ: Prentice-Hall.

Chinn, P., Winn, J., and Walters, R. (1978). *Two-way talking with parents of special children*. St. Louis: C. V. Mosby.

Condon, J., Jr. (1966). *Semantics and communication*. New York: MacMillan.

Glasser, W. (1965). *Reality therapy: A new approach to psychiatry*. New York: Harper and Row.

Leith, W. R. (1979). The shaping group: Habituating new behaviors in the stutterer. In N. J. Lass (Ed.), *Speech and language: Advances in basic research and practice* (Vol. 2). New York: Academic Press.

Leith, W. R. (1982). The shaping group: A group treatment procedure for the speech/language clinician. *Communication Disorders, 8*, 103–115.

Leith, W. R. (1984). *Handbook of clinical methods in communication disorders*. San Diego: College-Hill Press.

Meichenbaum, D. M. (1977). *Cognitive behavior modification: An integrative approach*. New York: Plenum.

Moore, G. P. (1964). *Organic voice disorders*. Englewood Cliffs NJ: Prentice-Hall.

Morris, H., and Spriesterbach, D. (1978). Appraisal of respiration and phonation. In F. Darley and D. Spriestersbach (Eds.), *Diagnostic methods in speech pathology* (pp. 200–212). New York: Harper and Row.

Murphy, A. T. (1964). *Functional voice disorders*. Englewood Cliffs, NJ: Prentice-Hall.

Pannbacker, M. (1984) Classification system of voice disorders: A review of the literature. *Language, Speech, and Hearing Services in the Schools, 15*(3), 169–174.

Perkins, W. (1971). *Speech pathology: An applied behavioral science*. St. Louis: C. V. Mosby.

Perkins, W., and Kent, R. (1986). *Functional anatomy of speech, language and hearing*. San Diego: College-Hill Press.

Van Riper, C. (1981). *Speech correction: Principles and methods*. Englewood Cliffs, NJ: Prentice-Hall.

Wilson, D. K. (1979). *Voice problems of children*. Baltimore: Williams & Wilkins.
Zemlin, W. R. (1981) *Speech and hearing science: Anatomy and physiology* (2nd ed). Englewood Cliffs, NJ: Prentice-Hall.

Index

—NOTES—

—NOTES—

—NOTES—

—NOTES—

—**NOTES**—